P9-DWY-601

CARING FOR YOUR OLDER
DOG

Chris C. Pinney, D.V.M.

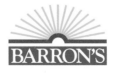

BARRON'S

Dedication

To Ubu, a grand old friend

© Copyright 1995 by Chris C. Pinney, D.V.M.

All rights reserved.
No part of this book may be reproduced in any form, by photostat, microfilm, xerography, or any other means, or incorporated into any information retrieval system, electronic or mechanical, without the written permission of the copyright owner.

All inquiries should be addressed to:
Barron's Educational Series, Inc.
250 Wireless Boulevard
Hauppauge, New York 11788

International Standard Book No. 0-8120-9149-3

Library of Congress Catalog Card No. 95-6756

Library of Congress Cataloging-in-Publication Data
Pinney, Chris C.
   Caring for your older dog / by Chris C. Pinney.
      p.   cm.
   Includes index.
   ISBN 0-8120-9149-3
   1. Dogs. 2. Dogs—Aging. 3. Dogs—Diseases.
4. Veterinary geriatrics. I. Title.
SF427.P57   1995
636.7′089′897—dc20   95-6756
                                                          CIP

Printed in Hong Kong

56789   9955   98765432

Acknowledgments

The author would like to thank M. D. Willard, D.V.M., MS, Diplomate ACVIM, and the College of Veterinary Medicine, Texas A&M University, for their valuable contributions to this book. Addi-tionally, a debt of gratitude is owed to my wife, Tracy, without whose support and patience this book would not have been possible.

About the Author

Chris C. Pinney, D.V.M., has written numerous books and articles about health care for pets and has hosted television and radio shows spotlighting pets and veterinary medicine. He continues to practice small animal medicine, with an emphasis on preventive and emergency care. He lives with his wife and three children in Schulenburg, Texas.

Photo Credits

The majority of the photographs in this book were taken by M. D. Willard, D.V.M. and the Biomedical Learning Resource Center, College of Veterinary Medicine, Texas A&M University. The photographs appearing on the following pages were taken by the author: 1, 2, 10, 12, 15, 23, 31, 32, 39, 166, and inside covers; Donna Coss: front and back covers; Dennis Dunleavy: 129; Gary Norsworthy, D.V.M.: 115.

Important Note

Always use caution and common sense whenever handling a dog, especially one that may be ill or injured. Employ proper restraint devices as necessary. In addition, if the information and procedures contained in this book differ in any way from your veterinarian's recommendations concerning your pet's health care, please consult him/her prior to their implementation. Finally, because each individual pet is unique, always consult your veterinarian before administering any type of treatment or medication to your pet.

Contents

Preface

Congratulations on your purchase of *Caring for Your Older Dog*. As a responsible dog owner, you have taken an important step toward a better understanding of the special needs of your senior companion. This book will guide you through the fundamentals of geriatrics—the study of aging and associated subjects—as it pertains to your dog.

Caring for Your Older Dog begins with a discussion of the effects of aging on the various biological systems and functions of the body. An important, practical chapter on preventive health care for older pets appears next. Included in its pages is information about nutrition, exercise, vaccinations, parasite control, grooming, and elective surgery for your elderly dog. Chapter 3 will help you better understand diagnostic procedures and interpret the laboratory tests that your veterinarian may need to perform on your pet.

In Chapter 4, *Caring for Your Older Dog* focuses on select diseases and disorders common in mature canines. The biological organ systems and associated diseases are presented, along with special diagnostics and treatments for each condition, where applicable. In addition, an in-depth discussion of neoplasia and cancer includes diagnostics and treatments for the various types of neoplastic conditions.

Chapter 5 of *Caring for Your Older Dog* continues the discussion of diseases and disorders in older dogs, with the focus here on clinical signs and symptoms often encountered. Handy etiologic listings allow for quick reference, and appropriate courses of action for each are discussed. Keep in mind that these differential listings are meant to be used only as guidelines, not as substitutes for your veterinarian's sound diagnostic protocols. Remember: The most effective treatment of any disease or disorder begins with a definitive diagnosis!

Would you know what to do if confronted with an emergency situation involving your pet? Chapter 6 offers practical first aid information that could save your dog's life one day.

Finally, *Caring for Your Older Dog* touches on a topic that can be uncomfortable to discuss: euthanasia. Although most dog owners shy away from this subject, an understanding of your pet's final days and what they may entail will ease the burden of responsibility, should a decision ever need to be made. When pain and suffering are intense, euthanasia may become your final act of love and kindness to an old, special friend.

There you have it! *Caring for Your Older Dog* is a comprehensive guide designed to improve the quality of life and the longevity of your older pet and to give you, the pet owner, a valuable source of veterinary information. Details of diseases or disorders not mentioned in this book can be garnered from the many fine texts dealing with health care for dogs available from your favorite bookstore or library.

If you are ready, let's get started!

Chapter One

The Aging Process and its Effects on Older Dogs

The rate at which aging occurs in dogs is dependent upon a number of factors. Breed size seems to play a major role in deciding the longevity of our canine companions. As Table 1 reveals, the aging process is inversely proportional to the size and weight of the dog; that is, small, light dogs age much more slowly than large, heavy ones. For instance, the average life expectancy of a Saint Bernard is seven years; that of a Chihuahua is 14 to 15 years.

Breed type also plays a role in the aging process. Clearly, certain breeds of dogs age more slowly than others. For instance, standard poodles seem to live exceptionally long in comparison with other breeds of similar size. Collies and boxers age faster and have, on the average, a shorter life span than others in their weight category. Another factor that can affect the life expectancy of dogs is the biological phenomenon known as hybrid vigor, which can occur when two purebred dogs of differing breeds mate and produce offspring.

Many of the offspring exhibit greater vigor and resistance to disease than either of the parents and often have a longer life span.

The care a dog receives throughout its life also has an important bearing on its longevity. For example, dogs that are fed table scraps and diets conducive to obesity can be expected to have shorter life spans than those fed well–balanced rations. Dogs that visit their veteri-

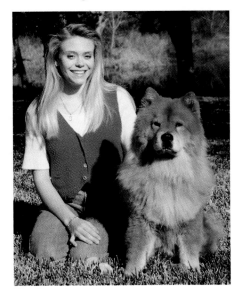

Table 1: Average Life Spans in Dogs*

Small breeds (1–20 pounds)	12–14 years
Medium breeds (21–50 pounds)	10–12 years
Large breeds (51–90 pounds)	8–10 years
Giant breeds (> 90 pounds)	7–8 years

* Oldest recorded age for a dog: 29 years

narians regularly and are kept current on their vaccinations, heartworm medication, parasite checks, and routine geriatric blood tests can be expected to live longer than dogs that lack such care. Finally, dogs that are kept exclusively outdoors tend to have shorter life spans, not only because of their greater exposure to adverse weather, disease, and automobiles, but also because they tend to receive less attention and nurturing from their owners.

Dogs age rapidly during the first two years of life, and the onset of puberty is early. With disease, predation, and exposure to the elements

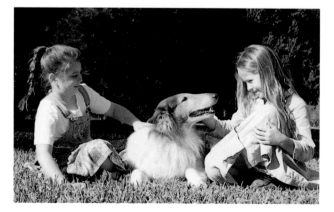

affecting the life span of the modern dog's wild ancestors, it is possible that early pubescence assured that breeding took place early in life, thereby ensuring propagation of the species. Further selection and refinement techniques practiced by professional breeders have resulted in some breeds' attaining puberty at six months of age!

After the first two years of life the aging process slows, only to accelerate again as the dog enters the final third of its life span. Many of the physical and mental changes associated with aging become readily noticeable during the last trimester of life. A touch of gray around the muzzle, a slight cloudiness of the eyes, and a slight stiffness in the gait are a few of the changes expected as a dog enters its senior years, changes that rarely warrant much ongoing attention from pet owners. In addition to these outward signs of aging, changes are also occurring internally, within the organ systems of the body, and they eventually will affect organ function. If impaired organs are not readily determined and subsequently supported through proper diet and medication, premature organ failure could significantly shorten the life span of a pet. How can these internal changes be monitored? Your veterinarian can provide the answer. Through regular checkups and appropriate preventive diagnostic tests, he or she can evaluate organ function within your dog's body and determine which, if any, supportive measures are necessary.

Now let's review some of the specific aging patterns that can be expected in the various organ systems as a dog advances in years and some of the management steps you, the pet owner, can implement to make your dog's life (and your own) easier.

The aging process is marked by a gradual decline in the rate of metabolism within a dog's body. In a broad sense, metabolism is defined as the aggregate of all the chemical activities within the body. These chemical reactions both consume energy and produce energy. If the body's metabolic rate is at its normal level, production and consumption of energy within the body will be in balance. Imbalances can occur, however, when the rate of metabolism slows during the aging process. The effects associated with a slowing metabolism include sluggishness, with an increased inclination to sleep; a growing intolerance to temperature fluctuations; and rapid tiring after exercise. A dog's immune system will also lose some of its effective-

Table 2: Comparison of Ages between Dog and Man	
Dog	**Human**
3 months	5 years
6 months	9 years
1 year	12 years
2 years	24 years
3 years	30 years
4 years	35 years
5 years	40 years
6 years	45 years
7 years	50 years
8 years	55 years
9 years	60 years
10 years	65 years
11 years	70 years
12 years	75 years
13 years	80 years
14 years	85 years
15 years	90 years

ness, and that creates an increased susceptibility to disease and an even greater need for you to keep your pet's vaccinations current. In a dog that is taking medications for long-term disease conditions, the ability of the body to break down and eliminate those drugs is also reduced with age, and periodic dosage adjustments are required as the pet matures. Finally, as metabolism slows, caloric needs decline as well. Appropriate dietary adjustments are in order, since failure to adjust your dog's feeding to these changing needs could lead to excessive weight gain and poor health.

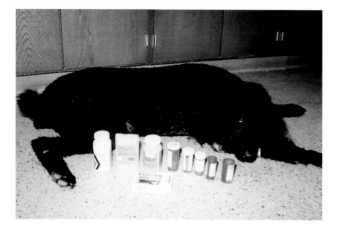

With age may come a host of health challenges.

Dogs do not suffer from atherosclerosis or "heart attacks" in the sense that we humans do, but they can be afflicted with diseases of the heart valves and heart muscle as they age. In fact, it is estimated that over 25 percent of dogs nine years of age or older suffer from some degree of heart disease. Further, cardiac output—the ability of the heart to pump blood throughout the body—drops with advancing age owing to normal wear and tear on the organ. That certainly contributes to the lethargy and exercise intolerance often seen in maturing canines. Dietary modifications, such as decreasing the amount of sodium in the ration, and special medications designed to increase cardiac efficiencies can counteract the effects of aging on the heart and blood vessels. Finally, inability to control body temperature may also arise as the blood vessels in the skin become less elastic and lose their ability to dilate and contract in response to temperature

fluctuations. To keep age-related stress to a minimum, take special care in attempting to maintain a relatively constant temperature and humidity in your pet's environment.

With increasing age, the capacity of the lungs to provide proper flow and exchange of oxygen to the body decreases. As with reduced cardiac output, lethargy and exercise intolerance result from the lowered oxygen levels within the body. Disease and scarring of the lung tissue in older dogs can also impair blood circulation within the lungs. That places an excessive burden on the heart, and leads to secondary heart disease and failure. Behavioral changes, nighttime confusion, and other signs of senility in dogs can often be attributed to a lack of oxygen in the brain as a result of poor lung or heart output.

The oxygen requirements of older pets must always be kept in mind. Clean, fresh, circulated air in your dog's environment helps to maximize respiratory efficiency. Second-hand cigarette smoke can pose a serious health risk to a pet suffering from a lung condition. In addition, excess humidity in an environment can adversely affect the rate of oxygen exchange within the lungs. Atmospheric filters and dehumidifiers should be considered, when applicable, to assist in oxygen delivery to the organs and tissues of elderly pets and to reduce associated stress.

As the digestive system ages, its efficiency in breaking down foodstuffs for absorption into the body is reduced. Periodontal disease (tooth and gum disease), which commonly affects older dogs, can lead to tooth loss. Routine veterinary dental checkups, in combination with at-home dental care, help to slow this progression and to preserve the important digestive function of the teeth. Further, the stomach and intestines of older dogs become much less tolerant of improper foods, such as table scraps. Flare-ups of gastritis and colitis can become commonplace, and dietary adjustments may be needed to combat bouts of diarrhea or constipation, as well as age-related dietary sensitivities. In addition, pancreatic and liver functions may decrease with age. That interferes with the conversion of foodstuffs to usable nutrients and makes it more difficult for the body to neutralize and eliminate toxic wastes. Enzyme supplements can sometimes help elderly dogs counteract such decreases in digestive efficiencies.

With advancing age, reduced blood flow to the kidneys creates scarring and other undesirable changes within those organs that disrupt their normal blood filtering and waste elimination capabilities. Subsequently, toxin and waste build-up in the bloodstream can lead to mental dullness, stomach ulcers, and other disturbances within the aging body. Feeding elderly dogs only high-quality diets and offering them clean (even filtered) water can help alleviate the

**Table 3:
Controllable Factors That
Can Adversely Affect
the Life Span of Your Pet**

- Obesity
- Feeding table scraps
- Feeding high-fat, low-fiber diets
- Keeping your pet outdoors
- Lack of attention
- Failure to neuter at a young age
- Failure to vaccinate
- Lack of preventive checkups

burden placed upon aging kidneys. In addition, good preventive dental care will help keep to a minimum the bacterial insult to the kidneys from this source.

Urinary incontinence, or inability to restrain urination, can also be a side effect of old age. Although usually related to loss of bladder sphincter control, incontinence can have other underlying causes as well, and this problem warrants a thorough diagnostic work-up. Incontinence in older pets may force pet owners to adopt new husbandry techniques to prevent complications associated with the condition. If your dog suffers from urinary incontinence, frequent bathing of the hair coat and skin surrounding the urethral opening is necessary to prevent scalding and irritation of the skin by voided urine. Keeping the hair shaved surrounding the vulvar opening of female dogs will also help prevent urine scalding. Finally, absorbent pads may be employed as bedding material to wick urine away from the skin of your sleeping dog.

As one might expect, fertility and reproductive performance in both the male and the female dog decline with advancing age. In addition, female dogs that are not spayed early in life are at high risk of developing mammary tumors and uterine infections as they enter their senior years. Male dogs that are not neutered at a young age will probably experience some degree of prostate enlargement. Left unnoticed, it could become cancerous and life-threatening. Neutering dogs prior to one year of age is the best way to prevent most reproductive problems. Dogs utilized for breeding purposes should be neutered as soon as their optimum reproductive life is complete (usually around eight years of age) or once you decide not to breed them any further, whichever comes first.

A decreased blood and oxygen flow to the brain, in combination with age-related degeneration of the nervous components of the senses (vision, hearing, smell, and taste) can lead to senile behavioral patterns in dogs over 10 years of age. These dogs become less and less tolerant to disruptions in normal daily routine as they mature. In addition, reactions to external stimuli become slower, and as senility intensifies, abnormal behaviors, such as poor recognition of familiar people and surroundings, poor appetite, and excretory indifference,

can result. Along the spinal column, degeneration of the disks located between the vertebrae can cause increased sensitivity to touch along the back and neck regions or weakness or lameness in the limbs. Often mistaken for arthritis, this condition can become debilitating if proper supportive measures are not timely.

As the pet owner, you can be supportive of these nervous system changes and sensory deficits in a number of ways if they affect your dog. For example, maintaining consistent and recognizable surroundings is important for dogs exhibiting any type of sensory compromise or senile changes. In addition, you may want to consider using invisible fencing devices or other means of "roping off" certain areas of the house or yard that may prove hazardous to a pet with such deficits. Remember to approach visually or mentally impaired canines slowly and audibly, to prevent startled and aggressive reactions. To adjust for diminished senses of smell and taste, warm your dog's ration prior to feeding; that will increase detectable aroma and palatability. Increasing your vocal pitch when speaking to your older pet can help compensate for diminished auditory function caused by nerve deafness. Finally, as far as changes related to the spinal column are concerned, older dogs, particularly those belonging to breeds predisposed to intervertebral disk disease, should be discouraged from excessive jumping and climbing, especially on and off furniture. Additionally, when picking up an elderly pet, always keep its back straight and supported to prevent undue stress on the spinal column.

Aging is also accompanied by a degeneration of the glands responsible for hormone production in the body. These hormones are essential to many vital processes of the body, and deficiencies or excesses of them can lead to a multitude of health problems. For example, hypothyroidism, diabetes mellitus, and Addison's disease are disease conditions caused by hormone deficiencies; Cushing's disease is marked by oversecretion of a certain hormone within the dog's body. All four of these conditions will be discussed in more detail in a later chapter. It goes without saying that routine blood tests designed to assess endocrine function in the aging pet should be performed at least once a year in dogs over 10 years of age.

As the support and locomotory system of the body, the bones, joints, and muscles experience tremendous levels of wear and tear during the normal life of a dog. As aging progresses, the cartilage lining the joint surfaces begins to split and fragment, and that leads to pain and arthritic conditions within the joints. A generalized thinning of bone throughout the body causes weakness in the overall skeletal structure. At the same time, excess bony deposits may be laid upon the spinal column and may be accom-panied by a deterioration of the cartilaginous disks located between the vertebrae. Both conditions can lead to pain and weakness along the back and in all four limbs. Additionally, loss of muscle mass in older dogs is a common phenomenon due to decreased activity levels, decreasing nerve function to the muscles, and excessive protein loss from the body. Loss in flexibility of the muscle tendons can lead to strains and injury in an overly active senior. Finally, muscle disorders caused by age-related disruptions in organ and gland function within the body can materialize in the older dog. Such disruptions, by causing toxin build-up or hormone-induced changes within the muscle tissue itself, lead to muscle pain, inflammation, and lameness.

There are several management techniques you can implement to help compensate for the musculoskeletal degeneration that may occur in your aging pet. For instance, keeping your dog's toenails trimmed short will help reduce wear and tear on the muscles and joints of the paws. Placing a carpet or throw rugs on slick floors in your house will allow a weakened dog to ambulate with greater ease and support. Also, providing ramps for the negotiation of steps or stairways will benefit animals with arthritic hips or back pain.

A generalized thinning of the hair coat, increased susceptibility of the skin to infection, and decreases in insulating capabilities are but three of the many changes that can affect the integument of dogs as they grow older. Abnormal proliferation of the sebaceous glands within the skin can lead to warty outgrowths called sebaceous adenomas or to the formation of nodular cysts (sebaceous cysts) beneath the skin surface. Fluctuations in the rate of skin cell growth and turnover, along with aberrations in the production of oily sebum by the sebaceous glands, can leave the skin of an elderly dog either too dry and flaky or excessively oily and greasy. Calluses may form on the elbows, lower hind legs, and other pressure points that contact hard surfaces.

The integument of older animals also becomes more susceptible to parasitic invasion by fleas, ticks, and mites. Stringent control of those pests is warranted. Allergies, which can afflict dogs of any age, tend to worsen with time. Finally, hormonal changes and internal organ malfunction caused by aging or by age-related diseases often manifest themselves as skin and hair coat disorders. For that reason, all dogs over six years of age that suffer from skin or hair coat disorders should have their blood hormone and enzyme levels checked.

Plan on brushing your elderly dog on a daily basis to promote normal sebaceous gland activity and hair turnover. Special attention should be given to flea control as well. In addition, proper precautions need to be taken if your pet is to be subjected to marked temperature fluctuations. Sweaters and cover-ups designed for dogs should be considered if exposure to extremely low temperatures is to occur. Conversely, if your dog is to be subjected to high environmental temperatures, it must be provided with a generous source of clean, fresh water and allowed unlimited access to shade.

As we have seen, the changes occurring in the body as a result of aging are complex and sometimes disheartening. The good news is that many of the conditions described above can be avoided or their impact lessened by understanding a few key points concerning husbandry practices and preventive health care for our senior canine companions. In the following chapters, you will learn in more detail how to improve the quality of life of your older pet and to ensure that its golden years are filled with health and happiness.

Chapter Two

Preventive Health Care for Older Dogs

Have you heard the cliché "An ounce of prevention is worth a pound of cure"? It certainly remains valid for senior dogs. A thorough plan for preventive and maintenance health care is essential to maintaining a high standard of health and quality of life for your mature pet. Many disease conditions and age-related changes in older dogs can be slowed or even prevented through the proper implementation of such a program. Focus areas in a well-balanced preventive health care program include nutrition and weight management, exercise, vaccinations, internal parasite control, external parasite control, regular grooming, dental care, and travel guidelines.

tional program include providing the highest level of nutrition and at the same time maintaining an ideal body weight, slowing the progression of disease and age-related changes, and reducing or eliminating the clinical manifestations of specific disease conditions. For instance, as your dog's metabolic rate slows and the tendency towards obesity increases with advancing age, increasing the amount of fiber and reducing the amount of fat in the diet can help keep the calories at bay and keep body weight constant (see A Word Concerning Obesity, p. 13). In addition, as the kidneys begin to lose

Preventive health care will help prevent your pet's medical record from looking like this one!

Nutrition for Your Older Dog

Once your pet reaches seven years of age, dietary changes are warranted to accommodate for the effects of aging and the wear and tear on the organ systems of the body. Goals of this senior nutri-

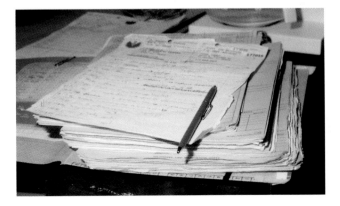

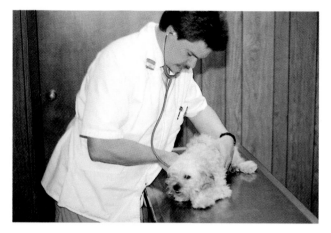

Regular veterinary checkups will help your pet live to a ripe old age.

their ability to handle the waste materials that must be removed from the body, dietary adjustments can play a major role in reducing the amounts of waste products the kidneys have to process. By reducing the sodium content of a ration, you can significantly lessen the workload placed on an aging heart. Finally, since older pets tend to have reduced sensory input (taste and smell), increasing the palatability of a diet can keep even the most finicky senior satisfied.

Here are some excellent guidelines to follow in feeding your older pet:

• If your dog is healthy, feed a high-quality ration formulated for the needs of healthy older dogs. As dogs enter their senior years, their caloric intake should be decreased by as much as 38 percent to accommodate changes in metabolism, assuming, of course, that they are not underweight to begin with. To help accomplish caloric control, these "senior"

rations typically contain more fiber and less fat than foods designed for younger dogs. Increases in fiber content also promote healthy bowel function in older pets. Because there are so many brands of senior formulas available on the market, narrow your choices by asking your veterinarian to recommend the brand that would best suit your dog.

Dogs suffering from specific illnesses need special diets prescribed by a veterinarian (see Table 4). For example, constipation, certain types of colitis, and diabetes mellitus often necessitate a fiber content greater than that found in standard "senior" formulas. In addition, older dogs suffering from chronic diarrhea, excessive gas production, or pancreatic problems can often benefit from special diets formulated to be more easily digestible than standard maintenance rations. Recommended dietary management of dogs suffering from heart or kidney disease includes diets low in sodium and restricted in protein. Last, older dogs that are underweight because of underlying disease may require a diet with increased caloric density to help reestablish their desired weight. Remember: Because these prescribed diets are so specialized, be sure to follow your veterinarian's directions for the amounts to feed and the frequency of feedings.

• Implement a regular daily program of moderate exercise for your dog

Table 4: Dietary Management of Disease in Older Dogs*

Disease	Dietary Adjustments Recommended
Allergy (food)	Replace existing protein source in ration with hypoallergenic protein sources such as lamb, chicken, or dried egg
Anemia	High protein/high-energy diet; multivitamin/ mineral supplement
Cachexia	High-protein/high-energy diet; multi-vitamin/mineral supplement
Colitis	High-fiber balanced diet
Constipation	Low-fat, high-fiber diet
Coprophagy	Low-fiber, low-fat diet
Cushing's disease	Low-fiber, low-fat diet
Diabetes mellitus	High-fiber diet
Diarrhea	Low-fiber, low fat-diet
Flatulence	Low-fiber, low-protein diet; soy-free; wheat-free; lactose-free
Heart Disease	Low-sodium diet
Kidney Disease	Low-protein, low-phosphorus, low-sodium diet
Liver Disease	Low-protein, low-sodium, low-fat diet
Obesity	Low-fat, high-fiber diet
Pancreatic insufficiency/ pancreatitis	Low-fiber, low-fat diet
Regurgitation	Low-fiber, low-fat diet
Urolithiasis	Low-protein, low-mineral diet; contains ingredients that maintain proper pH of the urine, depending upon the type of stones present
Vomiting	Low-fiber, low-fat diet

* Commercially prepared prescription diets are available from your veterinarian.

to promote weight control and to enhance digestive processes and normal bowel function.

• Weigh your dog monthly. That will afford an opportunity for early detection of significant body weight fluctuations. Such fluctuations could be indicators of overfeeding, improper ration selection, or the onset of underlying disease conditions.

• As for feeding table scraps and "junk" food to your older pet, don't do it! It only causes obesity and shortens life span. If you feel compelled to offer your dog treats during the day, consider using kibbles from a senior or low-fat ration as special rewards. To provide your dog with a satisfying variety, you can even use a brand of food other than the one you are currently feeding. Just remember that even such healthy snacks should account for no more than 5 percent of your pet's total daily caloric intake. In addition to kibbles, small portions of steamed vegetables can be used as low-calorie, satisfying treats.

- Be sure both food and water bowls are easily accessible to your pet, especially if it is experiencing diminished vision or arthritic limitations. Keep fresh, clean water available at all times. Remember that dogs suffering from kidney impairment or endocrine diseases such as diabetes may drink (and require) excessive amounts of

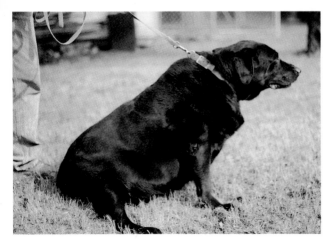

water; as a result, be sure the water bowl never runs dry.

- Vitamin and mineral supplements are rarely required if you are feeding your dog a veterinary-recommended ration. In fact, feeding such a supplement indiscriminately or inappropriately could lead to nutritional imbalances that might impair your pet's health. If you want to add to your pet's diet, consider using enzyme supplements in lieu of vitamin-mineral supplements. Commercially available enzyme supplements are thought to optimize the digestion of the rations that are normally fed, thereby naturally (rather than artificially) increasing the availability and intestinal absorption of proteins, fats, and carbohydrates, as well as vitamins and minerals such as zinc, selenium, and vitamin B6. Zinc, for example, is important to the immune system, and helps maintain skin integrity. Unfortunately, increasing the fiber content of older pets' rations can impede the absorption of zinc from the intestines. The enzyme supplement benefits your pet by extracting more zinc from its diet to offset the loss due to added fiber. Vitamin B6 is also important to a healthy immune system, yet significant amounts of this vitamin can be lost through aging or diseased kidneys. Again, increasing its availability in the ration will counteract some of that loss. Finally, selenium, a mineral that plays a role in the normal functioning of the thyroid gland, is also an important antioxidant, one that helps to counteract detrimental chemical reactions within the body that lead to aging. By freeing more selenium from the ration, enzyme supplements can promote thyroid function and fight the effects of aging.

Special enzyme supplements containing bromelain, a substance derived from pineapples, may have an additional benefit for older dogs. This enzyme, believed to have anti-inflammatory properties, either acts directly on the source of inflammation or promotes the release of nutrients and substances that are anti-inflammatory. Regardless of the mechanism, bromelain should be considered for dogs suffering from painful arthritis or chronic allergies.

- Besides enzymes, consider adding Omega-3 fatty acids to your pet's diet. Research has shown that these fatty acids, derived from cold-water fish oil, may effectively reduce inflammation caused by allergies and arthritis. Available from your local pet supply or pharmacy, these supplements should be dosed according to your veterinarian's recommendation for your dog's physical condition. Omega-3 fatty acids should not be given indiscriminately, since indiscriminately high dosages could have an adverse effect on the blood's ability to clot in the event of hemorrhage .

- As always, practice diligent preventive health care. That includes semiannual veterinary checkups to assess your pet's health and determine whether a dietary adjustment or change is warranted. Remember: Feeding the correct diet for your pet's specific needs will lengthen your years of companionship.

A Word Concerning Obesity

Keeping your dog's weight under control is one the most effective ways to add years to its life. Obesity can be defined as an increase in body fat resulting in an increase in body weight exceeding 10 percent of that standard for the dog's breed or body type. It is undoubtedly one of the most prevalent diseases of canine seniors today. Although obese dogs are not candidates for atherosclerosis and subsequent myocardial infarction, as obese humans would be, they are predisposed to a variety of other serious disorders such as hypertension, cardiac fatigue, pancreatitis, diabetes mellitus, and colitis. Skin disorders seem to be more prevalent in overweight dogs, as do disorders of the musculoskeletal and nervous systems, including intervertebral disk disease and osteoarthrosis. Simply put, obesity reduces the overall quality of life of these unfortunate pets afflicted with it.

The primary cause of obesity in dogs is imprudence on the part of owners who feed their pet too much food or the wrong types of

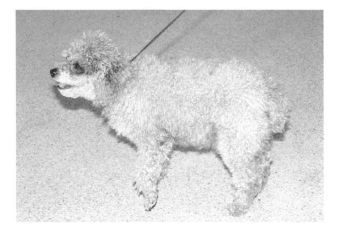

Exercising an elderly pet on a leash will help increase longevity.

food to. Among such foods are table scraps, a favorite of most ambitious canines. Owners who are swayed by big, sad eyes promote weight gain and create an annoying beggar. Failure to eliminate bad habits of this kind will lead to unprecedented weight gain as the overall metabolism slows with age.

Failure to adjust dietary requirements and amounts fed to a dog's age and specific needs is another predisposing cause of obesity. Senior dogs should be fed a diet consisting of one type of food only, unless treatment for a medical condition indicates otherwise. To counterbalance the effects of a slower metabolic rate, healthy seniors over seven years of age should be fed "less active" or "senior" diets containing higher fiber and fewer calories, rather than the regular adult maintenance rations.

If your dog is obese, simply cutting back on the amount fed will not provide the lasting weight loss you desire. In fact, depriving your dog of adequate amounts could create a state of malnutrition, leading to incessant begging and self-induced dietary indiscretions. The correct way to achieve weight loss through dietary adjustment is to feed your dog a ration that is specially formulated for that purpose. Such products are readily available from your veterinarian and should be used upon your clinician's recommendation. They generally have a high fiber content, which allows for caloric reduction while satisfying the hunger of your pet. Feed the amount recommended on the bag or can for your pet's ideal weight. If you don't know what that is, your veterinarian can assist you in making that determination. In addition, for added benefit and hunger abatement, divide the total daily ration into three or four feedings over the course of a day, instead of the standard one or two.

Along with dietary adjustments, exercise is a vital part of any weight control program. Following a thorough veterinary checkup, older dogs should be put on regular exercise schedules to promote fitness and weight control. (See Exercising for Longevity, page 15, for more information.)

Finally, not all cases of obesity in older dogs can be blamed on dietary indiscretion or lack of exercise. Hypothyroidism, a relatively common condition in older dogs, causes weight gain and lethargy. All obese dogs over six years of age should have a thyroid function test. If a problem is found, giving your pet a daily thyroid hormone supplement will assist in correcting the weight disorder (see Hypothyroidism, p. 82).

Exercising for Longevity

Incorporating a moderate exercise program into the daily routine of your older dog will yield multiple health benefits for your four-legged friend. Regular exercise, by increasing muscle tone and strength, will counteract some of the loss of muscle mass associated with aging. Exercise will give your dog greater agility and flexibility and loosen stiff joints. In addition, the benefits to heart and lung output are wonderful. Improved blood circulation, heart function, and lung capacities all increase your pet's quality of life and balance the ravages of time. Regular exercise will also promote and improve gastrointestinal motility, and that will stimulate nutrient absorption and help to prevent age-related constipation and anal sac disorders. Finally, keeping your dog physically fit during the golden years will help prevent obesity and its ramifications.

Before you implement an exercise program for your dog, a complete physical exam should be performed by your veterinarian to identify underlying health conditions that may limit the type and amount

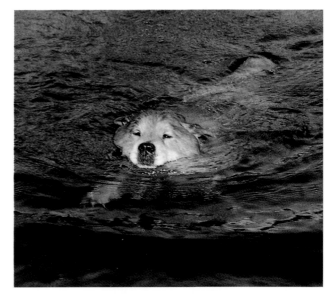

of exercise performed. In general, older dogs afflicted with arthritic joints and loss of muscle mass secondary to the aging process will decide for themselves what exercises they are willing to perform and how often they are willing to perform them. Dogs suffering from underlying heart disease may not be so self-regulatory, however, and could overexert themselves to the point of developing complications. Follow your veterinarian's advice closely in designing a fitness program for the needs of your pet.

Brisk walks on leash and leash-controlled swimming are the recommended modes of exercise for older dogs. Both provide outstanding results while minimizing the chances of injury. Additionally, the leash allows you direct control over the amount of exercise your pet receives. Swimming affords the

Swimming is an excellent form of exercise for older dogs.

additional benefit of relieving exercise-induced stress on sore and arthritic joints.

If your dog is out of shape, keep the initial exercise sessions short in duration and low in intensity. The ultimate goal is 15 to 20 minutes of brisk, continuous walking or swimming daily. Regardless of the type of exercise to be performed and your pet's physical condition, a five-minute warm-up period consisting of a slow-paced leash walk is critical to prepare stiff joints and to heighten cardiac output and blood circulation throughout the body. Once the warm-up is completed, the actual exercise session may begin. For best results when walking your dog on a leash, keep the pace moderate and consistent for the entire work-out period. There is no time for bathroom breaks; those needs should be taken care of in advance! If you choose swimming, you can control the amount and intensity of your pet's exercise by attaching a leash to its collar and guiding its swimming maneuvers. Fetching sticks or decoys thrown into the water can also contribute to the physical fitness of dogs that are willing to engage in such activities, provided the session lasts at least 15 minutes without interruption. Then a five-minute cool-down period, similar to the warm-up, should complete the session. Dogs opting to swim should be towel-dried thoroughly to prevent chilling.

During the exercise program of any dog over eight years of age,

watch closely for signs of overexertion or heart trouble, such as rapid tiring, coughing, and breathing difficulties. If those symptoms appear at any point during the exercise routine, immediately cease the activity. If your dog has not regained breathing composure within three to four minutes following cessation of exercise, contact your veterinarian.

After exercise, give your dog access to plenty of fresh water to allow for replacement of fluids lost during physical exertion. That is important, because in a dog suffering from even a mild degree of kidney impairment, failure to replenish lost fluids can result in dehydration and overt kidney failure. Isotonic sport drinks available in your local convenience store or grocery are also effective means; however, owing to their high sodium content, they should be used cautiously in dogs with cardiovascular (heart) disease.

Traveling with Your Older Dog

As one might expect, older dogs have special needs that must be taken into consideration whenever they are transported by car, plane, or rail, in order to reduce the chances of injury and stress-induced complications. In all cases, the safety and comfort of the passenger (and driver, when applicable) are foremost. You, as a responsible pet owner, can help achieve these goals by following a few basic travel guidelines.

First it is always advisable to use a travel carrier or kennel when transporting a pet by automobile. Your pet will feel more secure in a carrier, and that tends to reduce the stress associated with the ride. Moreover, it minimizes jostling and jolting movements that could prove quite painful to older dogs with arthritic joints. If your pet is too large to fit comfortably into one of these carriers, then the back seat is the place for it, not the front! The presence of a stressed-out, unrestrained pet in the passenger seat of an automobile is a liability.

Keep the inside of your car well vented and cool. Excited or stressed canines forced to travel in hot, stuffy cars or cars filled with cigarette or cigar smoke are likely to suffer ill effects. Tobacco smoke in itself can be quite irritating to the eyes, nose, and mucous membranes of an older dog and dangerous to seniors suffering from heart or lung disease. As a courtesy to your canine friend, refrain from smoking until you have reached your final destination. Car exhaust fumes can have the same effect as cigarette smoke. If stopped in traffic for any appreciable amount of time, crack the car windows and keep the air in the car circulating continuously.

As you have heard time and time again, never leave your dog in a parked car unattended for more than five minutes on days when environmental temperatures exceed 72°F or drop below 55°F. Keep in mind that older pets lose some of their ability to regulate body temperatures in response to environmental temperature fluctuations. As a result, they are more susceptible to heat stroke or hypothermia if left unattended in such conditions. If you have to leave your pet for a few minutes, be sure to leave two or more windows partially open to allow for air circulation. In addition, the use of window shields and sun visors is strongly recommended to help keep temperatures within the car at acceptable levels.

On lengthy trips, take along plenty of water, preferably filtered, for your dog to drink. Additionally, plan on making frequent "potty" stops along the way, especially if your dog is on any type of medication. Here is a useful tip: Freeze some water in a bowl prior to the trip. This "popsicle" can provide a long-lasting, refreshing source of water on extended trips.

If your dog has a tendency toward motion sickness, try feeding a small amount of food about 30 minutes before your trip. Often an empty stomach in combination with stress can predispose a pet to motion sickness. Never give your aging pet medication for anxiety or motion sickness unless it was specifically prescribed by your veterinarian. Tranquilizers and antihistamines, two common classes of drugs used for those purposes, can be harmful if given to a pet in an undiagnosed medical condition.

If you are planning to transport your elderly pet by airplane, extreme caution is necessary. Always consult your veterinarian beforehand to determine whether any medical conditions your pet may have could be exacerbated by such a trip. For example, high-altitude flying could prove harmful to a dog suffering from heart or lung disease. In addition, aged dogs too large to travel in the passenger compartment with their owner could be affected adversely by temperature and pressure fluctuations in cargo holds that would be well tolerated by younger dogs. Speak with an airline representative concerning accommodations for traveling pets; variations in policies do exist. Again, don't hesitate to ask pet health professionals for recommendations.

Finally, regardless of the mode of transportation, be sure to ascertain the location of an emergency veterinary hospital at your destination. If your pet should become ill during the trip, valuable time can be spared if that information is known in advance. Local phone books can be used as resources.

Vaccinations against Infectious Diseases

The immune system is a complex network of cells, organs, chemicals, and other molecules designed to protect the body against foreign invaders. One method of keeping this system primed for defensive action is the use of vaccines. Vaccines are preparations composed of one or more antigens, substances recognized as foreign by the body and capable of eliciting an immune response. The particular antigens used in the development of canine vaccines include specific viruses and bacteria that have been scientifically altered in such a way as to eliminate their ability to cause disease upon introduction into a host. Upon introduction, however, they will still stimulate special immune cells in the body, called B-lymphocytes, to produce specific proteins called antibodies. The antibodies, in turn, interact with and attach themselves to the foreign invaders, marking them for destruction by other immune cells and chemicals within the body.

Three basic types of vaccine preparations are utilized in veterinary medicine. First, killed (inactivated) vaccines contain disease entities that have been artificially processed and rendered noninfectious. Second, modified–live (attenuated) vaccines contain disease agents that have been rendered unable to produce clinical disease in the host. Unlike killed vaccines, however, they still have the ability to replicate within the host animal. Because of that feature, modified-live vaccines tend to stimulate a greater immune response than killed vaccines. The downside of using modified-live vaccines rests in the fact that there is a greater chance of causing a vaccine-induced disease if the vaccine was poorly manufactured or if the pet's immune system proves to be severely depressed. The third type often used, the subunit vaccine, consists of portions or pieces of actual disease agents that are noninfectious, yet have the ability to stimulate an effective immune response. Their advantage is that the immune response generated by the disease particles in the vaccine preparation provides immunity to the actual disease agent itself, thereby eliminating the need for use of the actual infective agent in the preparation.

As your dog matures, the importance of maintaining a current vaccination history increases. As with other organ systems, the function and efficacy of the canine immune system decline with advancing years. As a result, the immune response mounted against a foreign invader may be slowed or delayed just enough to allow the disease organism to gain a foothold within the body. For that reason, the aging immune system must be primed with regular annual vaccination boosters to help ensure the fastest reaction time possible.

The diseases your older dog should be vaccinated against yearly include canine distemper, canine parvovirus, canine infectious hepatitis, leptospirosis, parainfluenza and canine cough complex, and rabies.

Distemper

Effective vaccination programs have greatly reduced the incidence of canine distemper disease among the dog population in this country. This disease is caused by a virus related to the human measles virus. Because it can effect a multitude of organ systems at one time, clinical signs associated with canine distemper can be quite variable. Among those signs are coughing, breathing difficulties, eye and nose discharge, vomiting, diarrhea, blindness, and paralysis. Seizures that cause the dog to appear as if it is chewing gum are a unique sign of this disease. Dogs that survive an infection are usually left with permanent damage to their nervous system that may worsen with age.

Parvovirus

The canine parvovirus adversely affects the intestines and immune system of dogs. Spread through infective fecal matter, the parvovirus can result in a loss of appetite, profuse diarrhea, persistent vomiting, and immunosuppression that can quickly lead to dehydration, toxemia, secondary infections, and death. Because there is no specific treatment agent that will destroy the offender, preventive vaccination is critically important.

Infectious Canine Hepatitis

Infectious canine hepatitis is a viral disease that attacks primarily the liver, as well as other organs, including the eyes and kidneys.

Transmitted through the urine and other body fluids, it is characterized primarily by intense liver inflammation and interference with blood clotting. Associated clinical signs can include abdominal pain, jaundice, weakness due to internal bleeding, and a characteristic blue hue in one or both eyes. Again, no specific treatment exists to kill this virus once it gains a foothold.

Leptospirosis

Leptospirosis is a bacterial disease that can cause severe damage to the blood, liver, and kidneys. Transmitted from dog to dog through contaminated urine, the bacteria causing leptospirosis can cause fever, depression, vomiting, jaundice, bruising, and signs associated with kidney failure. Although this organism can be treated with special antibiotics, the damage caused to the organs prior to treatment may be irreversible. As a result, vaccination protection is important to stop this disease before it starts.

Parainfluenza and Canine Cough Complex

The parainfluenza virus, along with a number of other organisms, including the *Bordetella* bacterium, can cause severe tracheobronchitis in dogs. A highly contagious disease transmitted through infective respiratory droplets, canine cough is characterized by a dry, hacking cough that may last for weeks. Untreated dogs can suffer permanent damage to their respiratory systems (see Tracheobronchitis, p. 59).

Rabies

Rabies is certainly the most notorious of all diseases requiring vaccination. Characterized by hydrophobia and other symptoms associated with nervous system disease, such as seizures or paralysis, rabies is uniformly fatal to its unfortunate victims. In dogs, the disease is transmitted via saliva through bite wounds from other rabid animals, including dogs, bats, skunks, and a wide variety of additional wildlife. A definitive diagnosis of rabies can be achieved only through the microscopic examination of brain tissue from a deceased animal. Because of the potential threat to human health, most states require by law that a rabies vaccination booster be given on a yearly basis. (Note: Some states require a booster only every three years; however, because of the serious nature of the disease, this author recommends yearly vaccination.) To be legal, rabies vaccinations must be administered by licensed veterinarians.

Apart from vaccinations against the above-mentioned diseases, other specialized immunizations, such as that for Lyme disease, may be recommended by your veterinarian if you live in an area with a high incidence of those particular diseases.

To ensure that the vaccinations are administered properly and safely and that the vaccines have been stored and handled properly, utilize only the services of a licensed veterinarian when having your pet vaccinated. The health benefits to your dog and your peace of mind are well worth the extra cost!

Internal Parasite Control

To ensure that your old friend remains free of intestinal parasites such as roundworms, hookworms, and whipworms, stool checks should be performed every six months by your veterinarian. Early detection and treatment of worm infestations will help prevent malnutrition, diarrhea, and stress-related immune suppression from becoming established and complicating any pre-existing medical conditions. It will also lessen the risk of human exposure to these parasites, many of which can pose a significant health risk, especially to children.

Environmental management and cleanliness also play a key role in the prevention of internal parasites. Since fleas are the most common carriers of dog tapeworms, rigid flea control measures are essential to protect your dog against infestation by this type of worm. Further, daily disposal of fecal material deposited in your yard or near your pet's quarters by other dogs will effectively block transmission of infective parasite eggs.

If your dog is taking once-a-month heartworm preventive medication, additional protection against intestinal worms may be afforded, depending upon the type being given. Check the label of the heartworm preventive medication you are using to see if it affords such protection. If not, consider asking your veterinarian to switch your dog to one that does.

Dirofilaria immitis, the canine heartworm, is one of the most devastating and life-threatening enemies of dogs, both young and old. Its presence in a dog's body can put an incredible burden on the heart, blood vessels, and other organs, including the lungs, liver, and kidneys. In many cases, the concentration of these parasites becomes so great that affected dogs collapse and die suddenly. Transmitted from dog to dog by mosquitoes, heartworms pose a risk wherever and whenever those insects are found. Don't be fooled into thinking that the threat is eliminated just because your dog stays exclusively indoors. Have you ever seen a mosquito in your house? If you have, then your special friend is at risk!

Although the disease caused by these internal parasites can be deadly, the good news is that canine heartworm disease is completely and easily preventable through the use of heartworm preventive medications. Unfortunately, another myth that has been perpetuated among the pet-owning population is that once a dog reaches a certain age, the need for heartworm prevention diminishes. Nothing could be further from the truth!

Older dogs that contract this disease because of such neglect are not good candidates for treatment to rid their body of the heartworms, primarily because of the effect of the treatment regimen on a diseased or aging body. A pet may be forced to contend with the parasite within its heart for the remainder of its life, the quality and duration of which will be greatly reduced. The tragedy lies in the fact that prevention of canine heartworm disease is so easy and inexpensive. In fact, if your dog is not on a heartworm prevention program, call now and schedule an appointment with your veterinarian to start one. As a responsible pet owner, you owe it to your dog! In warmer climates where mosquitoes are present nearly year round, heartworm preventive needs to be given 12 months out of the year. In contrast, in regions that experience seasonal changes and cooler temperatures, preventive need not be given the entire year, but only during the warmer part of the mosquito season. Consult your veterinarian about the proper preventive schedule for your particular area.

Before you start a dog on heartworm preventive medication, have a simple blood test performed to determine whether exposure to this parasite has already occurred. If the test results are negative, then your dog may be started on a preventive. If they are positive, however, preventive medication is contraindicated. Giving such medication to a dog already harboring adult heartworms and heartworm larvae in its bloodstream could cause dangerous adverse reactions. Further, if you are giving your pet preventive medication and you miss a scheduled treatment, consult your veterinarian before resuming the treatments. Depending upon how late the treatment is, retesting may be necessary. Dogs on a seasonal prevention program should be retested before the first preventive of the season is given.

The most popular heartworm preventive medications come in either chewable or nonchewable tablet form and contain either ivermectin or milbemycin as the active ingredient. In the past, heartworm medication designed to be given daily was the only type of effective preventive available. Although the active ingredient of this daily preventive, diethylcarbamazine, is also quite effective at preventing heartworms if administered consistently, it falls far short of the overall ease and efficacy of the newer preventives. If you are currently giving your dog a daily pill, you should replace it with a once-a-month product. If you elect ivermectin for heartworm prevention in your older dog, use only the approved form of the product available from your veterinarian. Avoid using ivermectin preparations designed for cattle. These large animal formulations, available at some feedstores, are highly concentrated and could be toxic to your pet.

External Parasite Control

Fleas are the most common external parasites with which your older dog will have to contend. Not only can their bites produce extreme discomfort and even allergic reactions, fleas are also host to the most common tapeworm that affects dogs, *Dipylidium caninum*. Aging canines can be tormented by these pests, which may lodge on regions of the skin that an older dog is unable to bite or scratch on account of age-related inflexibility or arthritis. Further, aging dogs that are debilitated by disease seem to be prime targets for fleas. The exact reason is unknown; however, some think that changes in internal body chemistries due to disease or aging, or abnormalities in oily secretions from the skin may be to blame. Regardless of the cause, flea control is a vital part of any preventive health care program for your older pet.

The key to an effective flea control program is to first acquaint yourself with the life-style of this parasite. Its life cycle begins with the deposition of eggs both on the host pet and in the pet's environment, including both house and yard. Eggs laid on the skin and hair coat of the host usually fall off into the environment soon after deposition. In a house, fleas directly deposit their eggs onto carpeted areas. Other favorite sites include cracks and corners, damp floor-

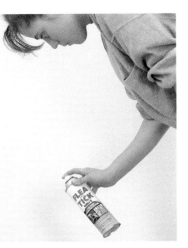

Environmental treatment for fleas is just as important as treating the pet itself.

boards and cupboards, and even air conditioning ducts. Of course, your pet's sleeping quarters will have their fair share of eggs as well. An adult flea lays three to 18 eggs at a time, and in her life span of a year she may lay over 200 eggs! The rate of egg laying increases proportionally with environmental temperature and humidity, and with the numbers of blood meals and male fleas available. Maturity of the eggs occurs most rapidly when the temperature is between 65°F (18°C) and 95°F (35°C) and the relative humidity is between 50 and 99 percent. In optimum conditions, the eggs hatch into larvae two to 14 days after being laid. The small white larvae that emerge from the eggs rely on adult flea excrement for food as they grow. Six months and three molts later, the larvae spin cocoons, in which they remain anywhere from one week to one year. It is important to know that while in the cocoon, the larvae are very resistant to

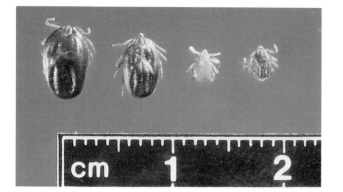

Controlling ticks is important not only for your pet's health, but for yours as well.

chemical insecticides and other environmental treatment modalities. Once fully mature adult fleas emerge from the cocoon, they diligently search out hosts upon which to feed. Incredibly, the average adult flea can live up to 58 days without food. Some species, after gorging themselves with blood, can live 200 days without another meal.

Another fact with a direct bearing on the effectiveness of your flea control program is that fleas, unless in the process of feeding, spend most of their time off your pet and in the environment, be it house or yard. Don't make the mistake of immediately discounting fleas as the cause of your dog's scratching just because you fail to observe a live specimen on its skin. Instead, suspect fleas whenever you notice chewing activity and see hair loss around your dog's hind legs and on its back, especially near the base of the tail. If you part the hair in these areas, you often will see the tiny black flecks of flea excrement that are left behind after feeding. That is a sure sign that you have visitors.

Because fleas spend so much of their time off your pet, thorough environmental treatment is necessary. Since there are so many products available, ask your veterinarian which flea remedies and protocols are safe and effective for your specific needs.

First, vacuum the carpets and floors of your house, as well as your pet's sleeping quarters, to remove as many eggs, cocoons, larvae, and adults as possible. Be sure to dispose of the vacuum bag afterward, since it will contain live fleas or flea larvae that could reinfest the environment through the vacuum cleaner if left in the bag. If a nondisposable bag is used, mothballs kept in the bag will kill any larvae or fleas collected. Next, after removing all people and pets, have your house (and your pet's house) exterminated by a professional exterminator. Alternatively, you yourself can spray, dust, or use a concentrated fogger containing an approved insecticide. Choose an insecticidal product with an ingredient statement listing an insect growth regulator such as methoprene or fenoxycarb. The combination of insecticide and growth regulator will eliminate not only adult fleas, but many of the larval forms as well.

The yard should be treated at the same time as the house, with any one of several products approved for this purpose. Chemicals most commonly used for this purpose include chlorpyrifos, malathion, and diazinon. Further, use or request products that are "microencapsulated" or that contain ultraviolet light-resistant insect growth regulators (such as fenoxycarb) for greater residual killing activity. For yards, use sprays or granules. To maintain flea-free premises, treatment of both house and yard with traditional insecticides should be repeated in 14 days, then again every three to four weeks during flea season.

In recent years, two notable advances have been made in the battle against fleas in the environment. The first was the introduction of polymerized borate compounds, available under various brand names from your veterinarian or favorite pet supply store. Sprinkled on the carpets and near the baseboards of your home, these electrostatically charged compounds will kill fleas upon contact. Noticeable results are usually obtained within one week. Best of all, the powder is odorless, easy to use, and safe for pets and children. Under normal conditions, the product must be applied every six to 12 months. Carpets must remain dry for continued efficacy; if the carpet becomes damp or is shampooed, reapplication becomes necessary.

The second advance is the use of beneficial nematodes to control fleas in the yard. Also available through your veterinarian or feed stores, these microscopic worms, when applied to a yard, eat every flea larva they can find! Harmless to grass, pets, and humans, beneficial nematodes are as natural a means of flea control as possible. Weather conditions and environmental temperatures will determine how often treatments must be repeated. Ask your veterinarian for more information regarding this new method of flea control.

When you treat your house and yard, treat your pet as well. The preparations for use on dogs come in the form of sprays and dusts, collars, shampoos and dips, and many other, less conventional, vehicles. For older dogs, the treatment of choice involves the frequent use of sprays. Sprays are preferred over powders or flea collars. If accidentally inhaled, flea powders can irritate your dog's airways. Flea collars rarely afford much flea control and may irritate the skin of older pets. Approved flea sprays, however, have two big advantages: They are safe and can be reapplied frequently. The sprays can be either alcohol-based—in which case they provide quick knock-down power— or water-based, for dogs with sensitive skin. The spray you choose should contain pyrethrins, potentiated pyrethrins, or pyrethroids (resmethrin, permethrin, d-transallethrin, fenvalerate, and the like) as the active ingredients. Rotenone, a chemical derived from derris root, can also be an effective choice. These chemicals are preferred over the stronger, more toxic insecticides such as organophosphates (chlorpyrifos, dichlorvos) and carbamates (carbaryl), because they are safe and efficacious if utilized properly.

Traditionally the biggest disadvantage of pyrethrin-type products was poor residual flea-fighting activity. With the development of "slow-release microencapsulation" technology, however, residual activity and subsequent efficacy have been dramatically improved. Whenever pyrethrin products are used, frequent spray application is imperative for effective flea control. In some instances it must be done on a daily basis. Whenever using an insecticidal product, follow label directions regarding frequencies and methods of application, and note any precautionary statements that may apply.

Along with flea sprays, shampoos and dips containing insecticide may be applied to your pet every two to four weeks to help control fleas. Shampoos containing pyrethrins or pyrethrin derivatives are the safest for older dogs. Remember, however, that shampooing your dog more than once every two weeks can lead to excessively dry skin; do so only on your veterinarian's recommendation. Flea dips are nothing more than highly concentrated preparations of insecticides. Chemicals such as pyrethrins, carbaryl, rotenone, and the stronger organophosphates are generally available in a dip formulation for use against external parasites. Remember, though, that misuse or misapplication of organophosphates can be harmful both to your pet and to yourself; exercise extreme caution in both preparation and application.

As always, confer with your veterinarian when choosing a shampoo and dip for your dog.

Insecticidal tablets and liquids designed to be taken internally (cythioate) or applied to the back of a dog for absorption into the body (fenthion) are also available through veterinarians. Since the active ingredients in these products may place undue stress on an aged or diseased liver, however, they are not recommended for dogs over eight years of age.

One of the newest products in the flea-control arsenal is a tablet containing the chemical lufenuron, an insect development inhibitor. This preventive, designed to be administered orally to healthy dogs once a month prevents flea eggs in the environment from hatching and thereby breaks the insect's life cycle. The intended long-term effect is elimination of the flea population in a contained environment. Lufenuron does not kill immature or adult fleas, however, nor does it kill an existing population of flea eggs or prevent other neighborhood animals from recontaminating an environment with fleas. Routine treatment of pets with topical sprays and yards with insecticides is still necessary.

Countless natural remedies for flea control have been touted as effective alternatives to chemicals. Many pet owners contend that products like brewer's yeast and garlic, taken in tablet form, are effective at warding off fleas. Unfortunately, controlled scientific studies indicate little or no benefit from these products. In addition, certain natural products containing abrasive ingredients (silica gel, diatomaceous earth) have been applied to the skin and coat of pets to control fleas. Those substances may dry or irritate your pet's skin, however, and their effectiveness is also questionable. Finally, many owners fit their pets with electronic flea collars in hope of controlling fleas without the use of pesticides. Although many manufacturers and some pet owners vouch for the effectiveness of such devices, research has demonstrated that their impact, like that of other natural remedies, is minimal.

After the flea, the next most prevalent external parasite affecting dogs is the tick. Controlling ticks on your dog and in your environment is important not only for your pet's health, but for yours as well. These unsightly parasites, which attach themselves to their host via sucking mouthparts, can transmit serious diseases such as Rocky Mountain spotted fever (RMSF), ehrlichiosis, and Lyme disease to pets and to humans. Both ehrlichiosis and RMSF are caused by bacterial organisms that can cause bleeding disorders, fever, swollen lymph nodes, pneumonia, and seizures in affected animals. Lyme disease, also caused by a bacterium, is characterized by high fever, swollen lymph nodes, swollen joints, and lameness. In addition to these diseases, untreated infestations can lead to skin irritation and, in severe cases, to blood loss anemia in dogs.

Female ticks lay their eggs in and under sheltered areas in the environment, such as wood stumps, rocks, and wall crevices. Once hatched, the larvae, called seed ticks, crawl up onto grass stems or bushes and attach themselves to a host animal as it passes by. Depending on their life cycle, immature ticks may seek out one to three different host animals to complete the maturation process.

Since ticks are sensitive to the same type of chemicals as fleas, treatment and control are basically the same. Thorough, consistent treatment of the yard and, if need be the house with an approved insecticide is the cornerstone of an effective control program. Since ticks can live for months in their habitat without a blood meal, treatment should be performed every two to four weeks (as with fleas) during the peak flea and tick seasons in your area. For your older dog, use a pyrethrin spray to kill any existing ticks attached to the skin and to discourage others from attaching themselves. Never attempt to remove ticks from your dog by applying manual pressure alone or by applying a hot match or needle to the tick's body. Most ticks killed by the application of a pyrethrin spray will fall off with time. In some cases, you may need to remove the dead tick manually after spraying. To prevent accidental exposure to disease, never use your bare hands to pick ticks off your pet. Instead, wear gloves and use tweezers to grasp the dead tick as close to its attachment site as possible, then pull straight up, maintaining constant tension. Once the tick is freed, wash the bite wound with soap and water, then apply a first aid cream or ointment to prevent infection. Again, be sure the tick is completely dead before removal; that will ensure that the tick's mouthparts remain attached to the rest of the body. If left behind, they can cause an irritating localized skin reaction.

Mange mites are microscopic parasites belonging to the same zoological class as spiders. They live within the skin or hair follicles of their host and feed on blood and cellular debris. Their presence often leads to intense itching, hair loss, and secondary skin infections. The most common types of mange affecting dogs are sarcoptic mange and demodectic mange.

For older dogs that are groomed regularly and are not allowed to roam the neighborhood, sarcoptic mange is rarely a problem. This type of mange is characterized by itching, hair loss, or thickened, wrinkled skin, especially around the dog's face, ear tips, elbows, thighs, and tail. It is primarily associated with young or stray dogs. Older dogs could conceivably become infested, however, through direct contact with a dog suffering from this particular mange mite.

Another common type of mite, the demodectic mange mite, resides within the hair follicles of dogs it infests, often causing secondary inflammation and infection. Demodex too is primarily a disease of younger dogs; it is rare in older dogs. Since a normally functioning immune system plays a key role in preventing this disease in both young and old dogs, diseases or drug therapies (cancer therapy, steroids) that tend to weaken or suppress the immune system could underlie an episode of demodectic mange in an older canine.

Diagnosis of mange can be made by your veterinarian by observing clinical signs and by examining skin scrapings obtained from your dog. Treatment for either type of mange employs special dips designed to kill the mites. In addition, treatment for demodectic mange may include the administration of ivermectin or milbemycin oxime (antiparasitic drugs), and antibiotics if a secondary skin infection is present.

Grooming Your Older Dog

Grooming is an important part of any preventive health care program. Not only will it help keep your dog in top shape physically, but the time spent with your old friend will provide your pet the psychological comfort that such interaction and attention create. As an added benefit, routine grooming and hands-on attention will assist in the early detection of external parasites, tumors, infections, or other changes or abnormalities that may result from the germination of an internal disease condition. The grooming program for your older pet should include skin and coat care (brushing, bathing), nail care, ear care, and dental care.

Brushing and Bathing

Regardless of the hair length of your dog, brushing its hair coat thoroughly on a daily basis will promote not only a healthy coat, but healthy skin as well. In dogs with exceptionally long or thick hair, twice-a-day brushing may be required, especially during the spring and fall months, when shedding is heaviest. Brushing with such frequency will help prevent tangles and mats and remove dead hair from the coat, paving the way for new hair growth. Brushing also stimulates sebaceous gland activity and blood circulation to the skin and removes skin scales and crusts that could lead to itching. The result of all these efforts will be skin that is moisturized and vibrant and a hair coat that is soft and shiny.

Be sure to choose the right type of brush for your pet's particular hair coat. As a general rule, the wider apart the bristles or pins are set on the brush, the longer the coat it is designed for use on. Combs can also come in handy if your dog has a fine, silky hair coat that is too delicate for conventional brushes. The teeth of combs, like the bristles or pins of brushes, are set at different widths for different types of coats: wide-spaced for thicker coats and closely spaced for longer, silkier hair.

When brushing, follow the grain of the hair and use firm, even strokes. If your dog has a thick undercoat, first brush that portion against the grain of the hair, then brush the outer coat with the grain. If you find a mat or a tangle, use your fingers to work as much of it free as you can, then gently run the brush or comb through it. If the mat fails to give way and your pet is experiencing discomfort as a result, stop immediately. Run electric shears close to the skin to eliminate such persistent mats. If you have no shears, run a comb as close to the skin as possible to entrap the mat on top; then, using scissors, cut the mat at the comb's upper surface. Never leave the skin unprotected when using scissors to remove a mat. Once the mat is gone, inspect the skin at that location to be sure it is not reddened or inflamed. If it appears to be only slightly irritated, it is likely to resolve on its own. However, if the skin is obviously infected or the area is severely reddened and inflamed, seek veterinary medical attention immediately. Remember: If you brush your older dog daily, there should be no mats and tangles!

As a rule, if you brush your dog on a daily basis the need for bathing is minimal. Routine bathing should be performed only for dogs that continually expose themselves to excessive dirt, grease, or other noxious substances in their environment and for canines suffering from external parasites or medical conditions such as infections and seborrhea of the skin.

If a general cleaning is desired for an otherwise healthy dog, it is best to purchase a mild hypoallergenic shampoo from your veterinarian or favorite pet supply store. Remember, though, that if your dog is afflicted with any type of medical condition, the. the type of shampoo should be recommended or prescribed by your veterinarian. For bacterial skin infections, shampoos containing benzoyl peroxide, chlorhexidine, or triclosan are generally employed. For seborrhea, shampoos that combine tar, sulfur, and salicylic acid seem to provide the best results. Oatmeal-containing shampoos are often prescribed for pets with itchy, allergic skin disease.

Before giving your dog a bath, brush its hair coat thoroughly to remove any mats and tangles. In addition, apply some type of protection to both eyes to prevent corneal burns if shampoo accidentally gets into the eyes. Mineral oil can be used for that purpose; however, a sterile ophthalmic ointment is preferable. Such an ointment can be purchased from your veterinarian or local pet store.

Nail Care

Because activity tends to decrease with age, the nails of older dogs experience less wear and consequently grow longer and faster than those of their younger, more active counterparts. Your dog's nails should be examined every three weeks and trimmed if necessary. Overgrown, neglected nails snag and tear easily, causing pain and discomfort. Additionally, nail overgrowth can lead to gait instability and joint stress, further complicating the life of older pets already suffering from arthritis or joint stiffness.

To determine whether your dog's nails are too long, look at the paws as they rest flat on the floor with your dog standing. Any nail that touches the floor surface is a candidate for trimming. Don't forget the dewclaws that may be present on the inside surface of the legs below the carpal (wrist) regions. Too often these nails go unnoticed and grow to exorbitant lengths in older dogs. Sometimes infections due to ingrowth are the result.

When trimming nails, use only a brand of nail clipper that is designed for pets. If your dog's nails are clear, you should be able to see the line of demarcation between the pink quick (the portion of the nail that contains the blood supply) and the remainder of the nail. With your clippers, snip off the latter portion just in front of the quick. For dogs with darker nails, use a flashlight or penlight beam to illuminate the quick prior to trimming. If that doesn't enable you to see the quick, snip off small portions at a time until the nail is no longer bearing weight. If bleeding occurs, stop trimming and consider having your veterinarian finish the job. Although ideally you want to avoid drawing blood when trimming your dog's nails, don't fret if some blood flows. Using a clean cloth or towel, apply direct pressure to the end of the bleeding nail for three to five minutes. In most cases that is all that is needed. For stubborn cases, apply commercially available clotting powder to the end of the nail to stop the hemorrhage.

Ear Care

Because the canine external ear canal is long and bending, routine care of the ears is needed to prevent accumulations of moisture, wax, and debris. That involves cleaning and drying the ears on a weekly basis and plucking any hair occluding the external ear opening. Many different types of ear cleansers and drying agents are readily available from pet stores, pet supply houses, and veterinary offices. Liquid ear cleansers are preferred to powders, since powders tend to saturate with moisture and trap it within the ear canal. Most liquid ear cleansers contain both a wax solvent and a drying agent (astringent) that clean the ear and dry it at the same time.

Before cleaning your dog's ears, look for signs of irritation, discharges, and foul odors. If one or more are found, your pet's ears should be examined by your veterinarian in lieu of cleaning. An ear

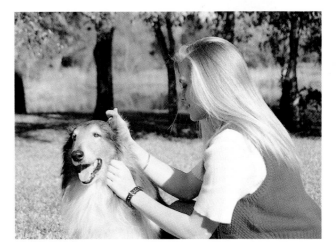

examination is recommended as well for dogs that appear to be constantly shaking or tilting their heads. Unhealthy ears may have torn or diseased eardrums, and introducing a cleansing solution can spread infection to the deeper portions and structures within the ear.

Assuming your dog's ears are healthy, begin cleaning by gently pulling the ear flap out and away from the head to expose and straighten the ear canal. Carefully squeeze a liberal amount of ear cleaning solution into the ear and massage the ear canal for 20 seconds. Next, allow your dog to shake its head, then follow the same procedure with the opposite ear. Once both ears have been treated, use cotton balls or swabs to remove any wax or debris found on the inside folds of the ear flap and the outer portions of the ear canal. To avoid serious injury to your dog's ear, never introduce the swab into the actual ear canal.

Ears should be inspected for inflammation and discharge.

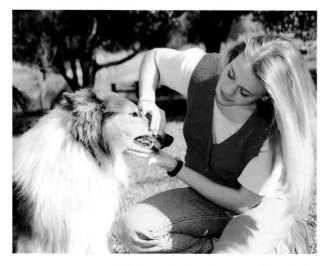

Keeping your dog's teeth free of plaque buildup will increase longevity.

Hair occluding the opening of the external ear canal can predispose the ear to inflammation and infection. Such hair needs to be removed or plucked periodically with tweezers or forceps. Again, if you perform an ear pluck at home, be sure not to insert your instrument into the actual ear canal. I recommend that ear plucks be performed only by veterinarians or experienced groomers. Plucking the ears can be a painful procedure, and it may elicit an aggressive response from your dog. In addition, plucking can lead to infection within an ear canal unless proper preventive medication is applied to the canal following the procedure. For those reasons alone, consider outsourcing this task to an experienced professional.

Dental Care

Keeping your dog's teeth free of tartar and plaque buildup is a preventive health care procedure that will add years to its life. It is estimated that tooth and gum disease (periodontal disease) strikes up to 80 percent of all dogs by three years of age. Not only do plaque-laden teeth and inflamed gums lead to halitosis (foul breath) and eventual tooth loss, but bacteria from these sources can enter the bloodstream and travel to the heart and kidneys, where they can set up an infection. In older dogs, infection of the heart valves and subsequent heart failure can all too often be traced to periodontal disease. Regular visits to your veterinarian for professional cleaning and polishing, supplemented by an at-home dental care program, are a must to keep your dog's teeth and heart healthy. (For more information on periodontal disease, see The Digestive System, p. 88.)

Because a short-acting sedative/anesthetic is required for professional cleaning, blood tests should be performed on your older dog prior to anesthesia to rule out underlying conditions that could complicate recovery. Fortunately, recent advances in veterinary anesthesiology and anesthetic agents have greatly increased the safety of this procedure in older dogs.

Once the dog is anesthetized, an ultrasonic scaler is used to shatter and break up the plaque that has accumulated on its teeth above and below the gumline. Then the mouth is rinsed and a polisher used on the teeth to restore their smooth, shiny surfaces. The entire procedure should take no more than 30 to 40 minutes, after which time your pet will be recovered from the anesthesia.

Professional teeth cleaning, as described above, may be required every four to six months. However, with diligent dental care provided daily by you at home, the interval between treatments can be extended to up to one year. Toothpastes and cleansing solutions designed for dogs are available from your veterinarian or local pet stores. For best results use preparations that contain chlorhexidine, an antimicrobial agent capable of hours of residual protection against bacteria that attempt to colonize the tooth and gum surfaces. Do not use toothpastes designed for humans; if swallowed, they can cause severe stomach upset in your dog. With soft-bristled toothbrush or cloth, gently massage the paste or solution onto the outer and, if possible, inner surfaces of the teeth and gums. If in doubt, ask your veterinarian to demonstrate the safe and correct procedure for brushing canine teeth. One at-home procedure not recommended here is routine teeth scaling using special dental instruments to remove plaque and tartar. Scaling should be performed only by a veterinarian, for two very good reasons. First, it produces small etches and grooves on tooth surfaces that, if not subsequently polished smooth, can act as nidi, or points where tartar and plaque can build up. Unfortunately, such polishing cannot be performed effectively or safely without sedation or anesthesia and special polishing instruments. Second, for maximum health benefit, plaque located on the portions of the teeth beneath the gumline must be scaled as well. As you might expect, that is a painful procedure, and to attempt it without anesthesia is dangerous to all parties!

Special devices that help keep your dog's teeth free of tartar can supplement brushing efforts at home. Certain rawhide, nylon, and urethane chew bones are specially designed to massage and clean a dog's teeth. In addition, commercially available flossing devices can reduce tartar build-up more effectively than brushing alone. Ask your pet health professional for details on these and other methods of keeping your aging dog's teeth and gums disease-free.

Periodontal disease is a leading cause of heart disease in older dogs.

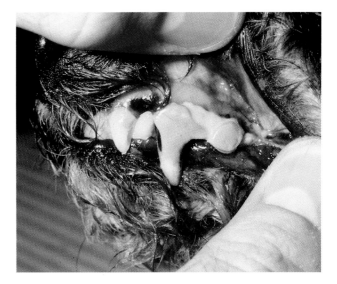

Neutering Your Older Pet

The term neutering refers to the removal of the ovaries and uterus (ovariohysterectomy) of the female dog or the testicles (castration) of the male. Because of the high incidence of reproductive disorders in later years, it is recommended that all dogs be neutered by their eighth birthday. Thus age-related uterine infections and pyometra in older females can be avoided and the incidence of prostate disorders in aging males greatly reduced. As an added benefit, female dogs that undergo this procedure before their second heat cycle are at less risk of developing mammary cancer later on than their non-neutered counterparts.

With proper preanesthetic blood tests and the use of only the newest, most technologically advanced anesthetic agents, the risks associated with such surgery in an older dog can be greatly reduced. The actual procedure should take no more than twenty-five minutes. Following postoperative recovery, a physical examination will be performed again before your pet goes home. Sutures are normally removed seven to 10 days after surgery.

Contrary to popular belief, neutering in itself is not a direct cause of obesity in dogs. Improper feeding practices, lack of exercise, and, in some instances, disease, are the causes, not reproductive status. Further, though neutering can have a calming effect on nervous or restless dogs, activity levels in emotionally stable dogs are rarely affected.

Sedation and Anesthesia in Older Dogs

Sedation and anesthesia are procedures that make it easier for veterinarians to perform certain diagnostics and treatments on older dogs. Sedation refers to the administration of an agent designed to alleviate distress, irritation, excitement, or pain. Its primary use in dogs is to enable diagnostic procedures such as radiology or endoscopy to be performed without struggle. Sedatives are also effective restraining agents for minor surgical procedures and for therapeutic measures not associated

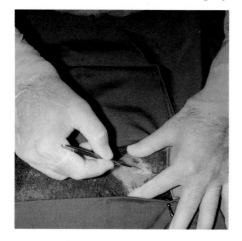

Having your dog neutered can help prevent a variety of old age-related diseases.

with intense pain. Anesthesia, on the other hand, is the induction of unconsciousness by means of an injectable drug or inhaled gas. Since dogs in a surgical plane of anesthesia are immune to pain, more invasive and extensive surgical and therapeutic procedures are possible. In many instances, sedatives are used in conjunction with general anesthetic agents to allow for easier administration of the latter.

There is no doubt that the risks associated with sedation and anesthesia are much greater in older dogs than in younger ones. However, with the advent of new, state-of-the-art sedative and anesthetic agents and the availability of new diagnostic technology to veterinarians, those risks can be reduced significantly. Before undergoing any sedation or anesthesia, your dog should be as healthy as possible, of course. A careful physical examination, along with a CBC, biochemistry profile, and urinalysis, should be performed before any agent is administered (see Chapter 3). That will help your veterinarian determine the anesthetic protocol best suited to your pet's condition and reduce the chance of any unexpected surprises. Food should be withheld for a minimum of twelve hours, water, for a minimum of four hours, before your pet undergoes anesthesia. Of course, exceptions to that rule may become necessary, but if an emergency arises, be sure to tell your veterinarian whether your dog has eaten or drunk water within these time periods.

Isoflurane is the newest, most technologically advanced form of inhalation anesthesia used in veterinary medicine today. A big advantage of this type of anesthesia is that only a very small portion of the agent undergoes metabolism in the body. The majority of it is exhaled from the lungs once administration of the gas has ceased. As a result, recovery from isoflurane is usually swift and uneventful. It is certainly the safest agent for older dogs, especially those with pre-existing medical conditions, including heart, liver, and kidney disease. Be sure to request it whenever your pet must undergo anesthesia for dental work or major surgery.

Chapter Three

Diagnosing Illness in Older Dogs and Interpreting Laboratory Data

When presented with an older pet that is exhibiting clinical signs of illness, your veterinarian will follow established diagnostic protocols in an effort to obtain a definitive diagnosis and select a proper treatment protocol. To save precious time in medical emergencies, nonspecific treatments may be initiated while the diagnostic database is being obtained.

First, your veterinarian will request a detailed, thorough history of your pet's problem, including, but not limited to, the time of onset, duration, frequency, and characteristics of the clinical sign(s). Accuracy is essential, since oftentimes this history alone can lead to a tentative diagnosis.

After a review of the history, a physical examination will be performed. Vital physiologic information, including weight, body temperature, pulse, and respiration, will usually be obtained first, followed by a systematic visual and hands-on exam starting at the nose and ending at the tip of the tail. The condition of the heart will be assessed with a stethoscope, and palpation of the chest, abdomen, and limbs will reveal any abnormalities or changes in anatomy and symmetry. Eyes and ears will be examined with specialized instruments. If clinical signs warrant more specialized testing of eye, nervous, and musculoskeletal reflexes and functions, it may be performed during the physical exam as well.

If the history and the physical examination fail to uncover the exact cause of your dog's clinical signs, further diagnostic testing will be needed. Oftentimes, financial considerations cause pet owners to forego further diagnostics and ask the veterinarian to treat the clinical signs instead of identifying and treating the underlying disease. Although a small percentage of pets will respond to that approach, most will not. Be prepared to trust and follow your veterinarian's advice.

Complete blood counts (CBC) and serum biochemical profiles performed on samples of your pet's blood provide valuable insights into the inner workings of the organ systems (see Tables 5–7). A CBC can be useful in diagnosing anemia, inflammatory and infectious diseases, and blood clotting disorders. Serum biochemistry profiles can identify increases or decreases in organ-specific enzymes, metabolic by-products, minerals, and electrolytes within the blood that may occur secondary to disease. Since most of these changes can be correlated with specific diseases, this analysis is invaluable in establishing a definitive diagnosis.

In addition to a generalized analysis of your dog's blood, laboratory analysis of its urine provides valuable clues to the cause of an illness. Kidney disease, liver disease, diabetes mellitus, bleeding disorders, and poisonings are some of the conditions that can be reflected in a urinalysis. Urine samples submitted for testing should be obtained at your veterinarian's office to ensure accurate results (see Table 8).

Microscopic examination of your pet's stool is almost always performed in a general diagnostic package, especially if your pet is exhibiting signs of gastrointestinal illness. Not only will such a test help reveal internal parasites that may be causing the illness, but the nature and content of the feces may be diagnostic for certain poisonings and dietary indiscretions. To ensure accurate results, your veterinarian needs the freshest sample possible. If you are unable to supply such a sample from your dog, your veterinarian can obtain one in the office.

Cytology, a newer diagnostic tool being utilized more and more by veterinarians, is the microscopic examination of fluids, discharges, lesions, or masses for cells and debris that may be characteristic of specific illnesses and conditions. The substance to be observed cytologically is obtained via a needle and syringe or a swab and applied to a microscope slide for special staining and preparation. Because of the importance and significance of this valuable diagnostic tool, veterinarians today are receiving extensive training in cytology in order to provide pet owners with state-of-the-art diagnostic technology.

One step up from cytology, biopsies are actual tissue samples removed from organs and structures by surgical or endoscopic methods. The samples are fixed in formalin, then prepared in the laboratory for microscopic viewing. Biopsies are especially useful in identifying and staging neoplasia in senior canines.

Radiographs, often incorrectly referred to as X rays, are pictorial representations of bones and internal organs. They are created by passing X ray radiation through a specific portion of the body that has been placed over special radiographic film. A portion of the X rays are fully or partially absorbed by the body structures, while others pass through unimpeded. That creates an outline image of the structure in question on the film, and this anatomical picture can be used for diagnostic purposes. Older dogs, especially those suffering from injury or illness, can be challenging to radiograph, since they rarely remain motionless while a radiograph is being taken. Sedation or anesthesia is often needed to provide the restraint needed for quality radiographs.

Radiographs by themselves may not provide enough anatomic detail to yield answers to your pet's problem. In these instances, special contrast materials such as barium or radiographic iodine may be administered orally or by enema, or they may be injected directly into a lesion. X rays are unable to penetrate these materials; as a result, they appear white on a radiograph, providing an excellent outline of the organ or lesion in question.

Another strategy that is becoming popular as an adjunct to radiographs is endoscopy, which entails the use of a special tool called an endoscope. This instrument consists of a long, narrow, flexible tube containing fiber optics and special channels that are attached to a light source and a magnifier. With an endoscope a veterinarian can examine most hollow organs, as well as body cavities, with minimal invasiveness and trauma. Endoscopes are commonly used to assess the overall health of an organ or cavity, to obtain biopsy samples, and to retrieve foreign objects from the respiratory and digestive tracts. In some cases endoscopy can provide an effective alternative to surgical intervention.

Ultrasonography is a diagnostic method that utilizes sound waves to outline internal organs and structures. Upon scanning a portion of the body, ultrasonic sound waves produce an image on a special screen that can be interpreted by a trained veterinarian. Ultrasonography is especially useful in identifying tumors within the body, as well as heart abnormalities. It is an excellent diagnostic tool, since it is simple, safe, and noninvasive.

Finally, exploratory surgery can be useful in diagnostics when all other tests and procedures have failed to reveal an answer. Although there certainly are inherent risks in using surgery as a diagnostic procedure, they must be weighed against the risks of failing to definitively diagnose an elusive disease condition. By performing a physical examination, CBC, biochemistry profile, and urinalysis before the surgery, veterinarians can assess a dog's inherent surgical risk and reduce it to a minimum.

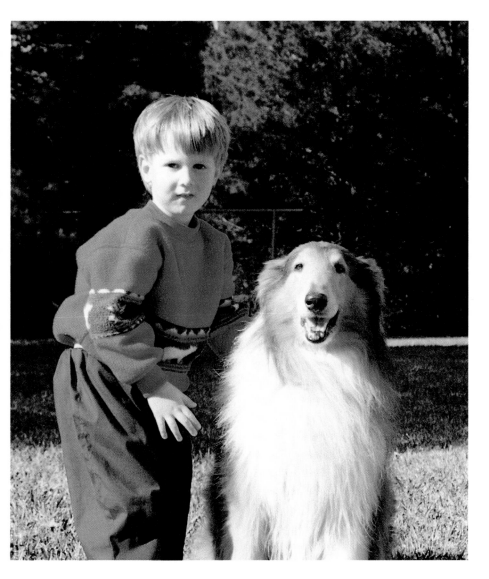

In addition to the above-mentioned diagnostic procedures, numerous other specialized tests can be employed in the event of an elusive diagnosis. Table 9 lists additional diagnostic tests that may be ordered if your dog is suffering from a less-than-obvious illness. Because each pet's condition is unique, the protocol and tests used by a veterinarian may not include those presented here.

Table 5: Components of a Complete Blood Count (CBC)

Hematocrit (Hct)
Hematocrit, or packed cell volume, is the ratio of red blood cells to total blood volume. Decreases in the hematocrit are caused by anemia, which can have several underlying sources; increases are seen with dehydration, chronic obstructive pulmonary disease, and, in some instances, hyper-adrenocorticism.

Red blood cell (RBC) count
Decreases in the red blood cell count are indicative of anemia, which can have several underlying causes. Increases in red blood cell numbers can be caused by dehydration. chronic obstructive pulmonary disease, and, in some instances, hyperadrenocorticism.

Hemoglobin (Hb) concentration
Hemoglobin is the molecule in red blood cells that is responsible for transport of oxygen molecules. Increases and decreases in Hb concentration usually follow those of Hct and RBC count.

Mean corpuscular volume (MCV)
MCV is the ratio of the Hct to the RBC count. Increases in MCV are caused by vitamin deficiencies; decreases are caused by iron deficiencies.

Mean corpuscular hemoglobin concentration (MCHC)
MCHC is the ratio of Hb concentration to the hematocrit. As with MCV, decreases in MCHC result from iron deficiencies and from an increase in reticulocyte counts. Increases in MCHC occur secondary to red blood cell destruction within the body.

Reticulocyte count
Reticulocytes are immature red blood cells that appear in response to ane-mia. A high reticulocyte count in the presence of anemia indicates that the body is attempting to replace the lost red blood cells. In contrast, a low reticulocyte count in the presence of anemia indicates that the body is unable, for whatever reason, to respond to the anemic state.

Blood smears and blood cell morphology
These smears, when stained and evaluated under the microscope, reveal size and shape abnormalities of red blood cells, white blood cell numbers and

types, and platelet counts. Red blood cell abnormalities can be caused by inflammation, neoplasia, or nutritional deficiencies.

White blood cell count

The total white blood cell count in a blood sample can help determine whether inflammation or infection is occurring within an individual. Increases in white blood cell numbers are usually seen with inflammation, infection, or neoplasia. Decreases in white blood cell numbers may occur with long-term, overwhelming infections, certain viral diseases, such as canine parvovirus, and poisoning.

White blood cell differentiation and percentages

Along with a total white blood cell count, a CBC will usually break down into percentages of total count the five different types of white blood cells. Neutrophils should make up the greatest percentage of white blood cells in a sample, followed by lymphocytes, monocytes, eosinophils, and basophils. Increases in neutrophil numbers are seen with stress, excitement, inflammation, infections with bacteria, fungi, or viruses, parasitic infestations, tissue damage, neoplasia, and autoimmune disease. Decreases may be indicative of a severe bacterial infection, certain viral infections, such as canine parvovirus, toxins, and bone marrow disorders. Lymphocyte percentages can increase with ehrlichiosis (a parasitic disease of dogs), allergies, autoimmune disease, Addison's disease, and leukemia, or following routine vaccinations. Declines in lymphocyte counts can occur secondary to endocrine diseases, such as Cushing's disease, chemotherapy for neoplasia, chylothorax, or any long-standing, stressful disease or disorder. Monocyte levels increase with chronic infections, heartworms, fungal diseases, autoimmune disease, trauma, stress, and neoplasia. Decreases in monocyte numbers are not clinically significant. Elevations in eosinophil numbers in older dogs are usually seen with parasitic infestations, allergies, and tumors, while decreases occur secondarily to stress and early inflammation or infection. Finally, basophils are rarely found in the bloodstream, and their presence can be indicative of heartworm disease, allergic skin disease, neoplasia, Cushing's disease, or hypothyroidism.

Platelet count

Platelets serve a vital role in the body's blood clotting mechanism. Decreases in platelet numbers, or interference with their function can lead to uncontrolled hemorrhage. Decreases in the number of platelets in any given blood sample result from autoimmune disease, excessive consumption due to internal bleeding or clotting, chemotherapy, and bone marrow disorders.

Table 6: Components of a Biochemical Profile and Their Interpretation

Blood urea nitrogen (BUN)
Blood urea nitrogen is a by-product of protein metabolism within the body. Increases in BUN can be caused by dehydration, kidney disease, cardiovascular disease, and shock. Decreases in BUN can be seen in liver disease.

Serum creatinine
Creatinine is a compound made from amino acids. The amount of creatinine in the blood is closely regulated by the kidneys. As a result, abnormal elevations of this substance in the blood are indicative of kidney disease.

Glucose
Glucose is the sugar which is the primary source of energy within the body. Marked increases in the glucose content of the blood can occur with diabetes mellitus, Cushing's disease, stress, drug therapy, convulsions, and excitement, and within hours after a meal. Decreases in glucose levels can be seen with liver disease, advanced seizure activity, Addison's disease, gastrointestinal disease, parasitism, starvation, and neoplasia.

Sodium
This chemical element is important to the fluid balance within the body. Increases in sodium are caused by dehydration and high fever. Decreases are seen in Addison's disease, vomiting, diarrhea, starvation, kidney disease, diabetes mellitus, and bladder disease.

Potassium
Potassium is another chemical element found within the body. Increases in potassium levels are seen with kidney disease, Addison's disease, tissue damage, and dehydration. Diminished amounts of potassium in the blood occur secondarily to vomiting, diarrhea, Cushing's disease, drug therapy (insulin, diuretics), and malnutrition.

Chloride
Chloride is a salt within the body that is also important to the water and pH balance within the body. Increases can be caused by diarrhea, kidney disease, diabetes mellitus, and shock. Decreases in chloride levels occur secondarily to vomiting, diarrhea, malnutrition, and diabetes insipidus.

Calcium
The most abundant mineral within the body, calcium is important for muscle function, heart function, blood clotting, nerve conduction, and integrity of the teeth and bones. Tumors, hyperparathyroidism, Addison's disease, bone infections, and kidney failure can cause increases in blood calcium levels. Decreases in calcium levels are seen with pancreatitis and low blood protein levels.

Phosphorus
This chemical element helps run important metabolic processes throughout the body. It also contributes to the structural integrity of bone. Elevations are seen with bone tumors, kidney disease, and hypoparathyroidism. Decreases are caused by hyperparathyroidism, tumors, and poor nutrition.

Total serum protein
Total serum protein levels refer to levels of albumin, which is a transport protein within the blood, and globulin proteins, which are important for transporting substances in the blood and for immunity. Increases in total protein levels result from dehydration and immune responses to infection. Decreases in serum protein are seen with immunodeficiency disease, gastrointestinal disease, parasitism, pancreatic disease, liver disease, kidney disease, blood loss, Addison's disease, and severe skin disease.

Creatinine phosphokinase (CPK)
Not to be confused with serum creatinine, CPK is an enzyme found primarily in muscle and brain tissue. Elevations in this enzyme occur with muscle disease and trauma.

Lactic dehydrogenase (LDH)
LDH is an enzyme found in the cell membranes of most tissues, especially the kidneys, muscle, and liver. Serum elevations are seen with muscle disease, liver disease, heart disease, red blood cell destruction, and tissue necrosis.

Asparate aminotransferase (AST, SGOT)
This enzyme is found in tissues throughout the body, including the heart, liver, muscle, and blood. Increases in AST are caused by liver, heart, and muscle disease.

Alanine aminotransferase (ALT, SGPT)
ALT is a liver-specific enzyme. As a result, elevations in this enzyme are indicative of liver disease, specifically damage to the liver tissue itself.

Alkaline phosphatase (ALP, SAP)

Alkaline phosphatase is an enzyme found on cell membranes throughout the body. Elevations of this substance are most commonly seen with liver disease, Cushing's disease, steroid drug therapy, hyperparathyroidism, and neoplasia.

Bilirubin

Bilirubin is a pigment found in blood and in bile. Produced by the liver, originates in the breakdown of the oxygen-carrying molecules found in red blood cells (hemoglobin) and muscle tissue (myoglobin). Increases are seen in liver disease, red blood cell destruction, muscle disease and trauma.

Bile acids

These compounds are derived from cholesterol and produced in the liver. They are responsible for the absorption of fat from the small intestine. Abnormalities in the amount of bile acids detected in the bloodstream are indicative of liver disease.

Cholesterol

Cholesterol, a steroid compound produced primarily by the liver, is vital to normal cellular structure and function. Increases occur with kidney disease, hypothyroidism, liver disease, Cushing's disease, gastrointestinal disease, diabetes mellitus, and pancreatitis. Decreases in normal levels usually occur because of improper fat digestion.

Gamma Glutamyltransferase (GGT)

GGT is found in the liver, kidney, and pancreas. Elevations in this enzyme are usually attributable to liver disease, steroid drug therapy, or treatment with anticonvulsant medications.

Amylase

Amylase, an enzyme produced in the pancreas, is also found in the liver and intestinal lining. It functions in the normal digestion of nutrients. Elevations are seen with pancreatic disease, kidney failure, Cushing's disease, liver disease, and gastrointestinal disease.

Lipase

Lipase is an enzyme produced by the pancreas and by the lining of the stomach. Increases in serum levels can be caused by pancreatic disease, kidney failure, Cushing's disease, liver disease, and gastrointestinal disease.

Table 7: Correlation of Clinical Disease with Biochemical Changes

Disease Condition	Look for Changes in:
Kidney disease	BUN Serum creatinine Sodium Potassium Phosphorus Calcium
Liver disease	ALT AST ALP GGT Bilirubin Bile Acids Glucose Cholesterol
Adrenal gland disease	ALP ALT AST Glucose Cholesterol Sodium Potassium Phosphorus Calcium
Muscle disease	CPK AST LDH Bilirubin
Pancreatic disease	Amylase Lipase
Bone disease	Calcium Phosphorus

Volume

In older dogs, the volume of urine produced is important information if kidney disease is suspected. In dogs suffering from actual kidney failure, urine volume is an important parameter in the determination of a prognosis.

Color and appearance

Normal urine is yellow to amber in color, the intensity of which depends upon water content. Dogs that are dehydrated have dark yellow urine as the body attempts to conserve water. In contrast, urine that is so light in color that it resembles water may simply indicate overhydration or more serious, it could indicate that the kidneys are unable to concentrate the urine with filtered wastes. Urine that is red in appearance contains blood. Orange-colored or brown urine may also indicate the presence of blood, as well as hemoglobin or myoglobin, the latter of which shows up as the result of muscle trauma. Greenish urine is seen with increased amounts of bilirubin or with certain bacterial infections. Finally, normal urine is clear and transparent to the naked eye. Cloudy urine can be seen with increased amounts of blood cells, bacteria, fungi, mucous, spermatozoa and prostatic fluid, and crystals.

Specific gravity

Specific gravity reflects the amount and weight of substances found in the urine. As the kidneys concentrate the urine with waste material, specific gravity should increase. In addition, dehydration normally causes an increase in this parameter. Low specific gravity, indicating dilute urine, in itself does not necessarily mean that disease is present; however, repeated readings of a low specific gravity in combination with dehydration usually means that kidney disease is present. In addition, other disease conditions that can cause a low urine specific gravity include diabetes insipidus, liver disease, Cushing's disease, diabetes mellitus, and pyometra.

pH

The pH of a dog's urine is normally acidic. Alkaline urine with a pH above 7.5 is usually indicative of a urinary tract infection or bacterial contamination of the urine sample. It is important to note, however, that bacterial infections can exist in an acidic pH as well.

Protein
Under normal conditions, the urine of a dog contains only trace amounts of protein. Any measurable increases can be due to kidney disease, hemoglobin or myoglobin in the urine, inflammatory debris, and blood cells.

Glucose
Glucose is measurable in the urine of healthy dogs. Glucose in the urine is most often caused by diabetes mellitus. Other etiologies can include pancreatitis, Cushing's disease, kidney failure, and certain tumors.

Ketones
Ketones are formed when abnormalities in fat and energy metabolism occur; as a result, they should not be found in the urine of normal dogs. Persistent fever, starvation, and diabetes mellitus can lead to the appearance of ketones in the urine.

Occult blood
The presence of occult blood in the urine indicates the presence of red blood cells, hemoglobin, or myoglobin.

White blood cells
Although the results of this test may be less than reliable, the presence of white blood cells in the urine is indicative of a urinary tract infection.

Bilirubin
Bilirubin may be present in trace amounts in the urine of healthy dogs. However, elevated amounts indicate red blood cell destruction within the body or liver disease.

Urine sediment
Microscopic analysis of the sediment formed by centrifuging a urine sample is useful in identifying white blood cells, red blood cells, bacteria, urinary crystals, casts, and epithelial cells. Urinary crystals often form as a result of a urinary tract infection. Casts are cylindrical accumulations of cells or debris that occur secondary to kidney disease. Finally, abnormal amounts of epithelial cells from the kidneys or bladder are indicative of inflammation, infection, or neoplasia affecting those organs

---

Table 9: Specialized Diagnostic Tests Utilized in Veterinary Medicine

Diagnostic Test	Target System/Group Tests For This Problem
Cardiovascular and pulmonary system	
Heartworm antigen test	Canine heartworm disease
Electrocardiogram (ECG)	Abnormal electrical activity within the heart
Bleeding profile	Blood clotting disorders
Blood gas profile	pH imbalances within the body
Angiogram	Circulation disturbances
Bone marrow analysis	Abnormalities in the production of blood cells
Urinary and reproductive systems	
Endogenous creatinine clearance test	Abnormalities in kidney filtration rates
Vaginal/prostatic flush and cytology	Infections, tumors
Musculoskeletal system	
Electromyogram (EMG)	Abnormal muscle activity
Joint cytology/cultures	Arthritis
Nervous system	
Electroencephalogram (EEG)	Abnormal electrical activity within the brain
Neurologic examination	Abnormalities in neurologic reflex activity
Cerebrospinal fluid analysis/culture	Infectious diseases; inflammation
Myelogram	Degenerative disk disease; spinal cord disorders
Magnetic resonance imaging (MRI)	Brain or spinal cord lesions
Computed tomography (CT scan)	Brain or spinal cord lesions
Endocrine system	
Thyroid hormone profile (T3,T4, TSH stimulation)	Hypothyroidism
ACTH stimulation test/ plasma ACTH concentrations	Cushing's disease, Addison's disease

| Insulin/glucose ratio | Diabetes mellitus |
| ADH response test | Diabetes insipidus |

Gastrointestinal system

Fecal trypsin test	Poor fat digestion
Food allergy trial	Food allergies
BT-PABA test	Pancreatic disease
Xylose absorption test	Intestinal disease
Sudan/iodine staining of feces	Pancreatic disease

Skin and hair coat

Skin scrape	Mange mites
Dermatophyte test medium (DTM)	Ringworm
Thyroid hormone assay	Hypothyroidism
Allergy testing	Specific skin allergies
Autoimmune profile	Autoimmune skin diseases

Immune system

Antinuclear antibody (ANA) test	Autoimmune disease
Lupus erythematosus (LE) test	Autoimmune disease
Rheumatoid factor	Autoimmune disease
Bone marrow analysis	Abnormalities in the production of immune cells

Eyes

Schirmer tear test	Keratoconjunctivitis sicca
Tonometry	Glaucoma
Electroretinogram (ERG)	Abnormalities in retinal function
Corneal staining	Ulcers on the cornea

Infectious diseases

Serum antigen tests	Specific disease agents (such as parvovirus)
Antibody titers	Antibodies to specific disease agents
Culture/sensitivity	Specific organisms/sensitivity to drugs

Chapter Four

Select Diseases and Disorders Affecting the Body Systems of Older Dogs

N ow it is time to focus attention on select illnesses that are common in older dogs. The conditions described here are only a few of the many geriatric diseases and disorders. A proper diagnostic protocol performed by a qualified veterinarian is still essential to ensure proper identification of any illness.

The Cardiovascular and Hemolymphatic Systems

The function of the cardiovascular system is to transport oxygen and nutrients to, and carbon dioxide and waste material from, tissues and organs throughout the body. At the center of this system is the heart, a hollow organ with strong, muscular walls. Valves within those walls keep blood flowing efficiently in one direction. Heart murmurs, often heard in dogs suffering from congestive heart failure, are caused by the backflow or regurgitation of blood through diseased heart valves. From the heart, thick-walled, elastic arteries carry oxygen-rich blood to the tissues of the body. After an exchange of oxygen, nutrients, or wastes has taken place, thin-walled veins carry the blood back to the heart.

The cells that make up the blood itself include leukocytes (white blood cells), a front line of defense against infections and foreign invaders; tiny cell fragments called platelets, which are required for proper blood clotting; and erythrocytes (red blood cells), which transport oxygen. Hemoglobin is the molecule within red blood cells that enables the cell to carry oxygen to the tissues. The noncellular portion of the blood contains water, nutrients, waste products, blood clotting factors, and a wide variety of hormones, enzymes, plasma proteins, and electrolytes.

In addition to blood, a liquid material called lymph is circulated in the body. This fluid contains immune cells (lymphocytes), proteins, and fat absorbed from the body tissues and from the intestinal tract. It is conveyed by special lymphatic vessels through rhythmical contractions associated with normal breathing and muscular activity. Eventually, after passing through many lymph nodes, which remove foreign substances and organisms from the fluid, the lymph reaches the bloodstream and reenters general circulation. In older dogs, edema, or fluid retention within the tissues, can be caused by tumors or other disorders that block the normal flow of lymph through the lymphatic vessels.

Heart Disease and Heart Failure

Of all the diseases affecting older dogs, heart disease and heart failure are among the most common. Heart failure is characterized by a decrease in cardiac output and a corresponding increase in blood pressure. For instance, if the left ventricle of the heart fails to pump blood properly, blood pressure rises within the vessels in the lungs. That leads to fluid accumulation within the lungs (congestive heart failure) and reduced exchange of oxygen. If the right ventricle is involved, pressure rises in the vessels throughout

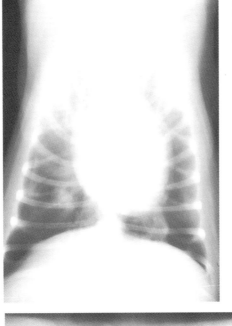

Enlarged heart associated with heart disease.

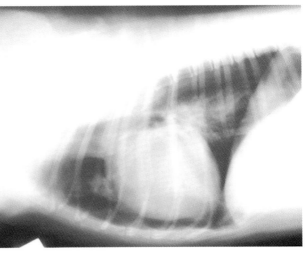

the body and causes tissue swelling and fluid buildup within the abdomen (ascites).

The most common type of heart failure in older dogs is mitral insufficiency, characterized by a deteriora-

51

tion of the mitral valve, located in the left side of the heart. Deterioration causes the valve to close improperly, so that a backflow of blood occurs upon contraction. As a result the amount of blood circulated with each heart contraction is reduced, and that leads to increased blood pressure within the vessels returning from the lungs.

Deterioration of the mitral valve may be a function of age or, more important, a result of bacterial infection and associated inflammation of the valve itself. Bacteria from infected teeth and gums can enter the bloodstream and attach themselves to the mitral valve. Over time the heart valve itself becomes damaged and scarred by this infection, and its normal function is disrupted.

Although their frequency of occurrence is lower, diseases involving the other valves in the heart do occur. For example, disease of the tricuspid valve, located in the right side of the heart, can also occur secondary to aging or to infection, and it can interfere with the normal return of blood to the heart from the body. When that happens, ascites and an enlarged abdomen can result. In addition, defects in other valves of the heart can be congenital (present at birth) in nature and may not be detectable until the dog grows older and the work load placed on the heart increases.

Valvular disease is not the only cause of heart failure in older dogs. Cardiomyopathy, or disease of the heart muscle itself, can also lead to failure of this organ. Cardiomyopathy has two forms: dilative cardiomyopathy, characterized by a thinning of the wall of the heart, and hypertrophic cardiomyopathy, characterized by an abnormal enlargement and thickening of the heart muscle. Regardless of the type, cardiomyopathies interfere with the normal contractility of the heart and lead to eventual heart failure.

Arrhythmias, or deviations from the normal rate or rhythm of the actual heartbeat, are additional disorders of heart function in older dogs. When arrhythmias occur, the heart muscle either fails to contract in the proper sequence or contracts too quickly or too slowly. In any case, poor blood circulation results. Two potential causes of arrhythmias in older dogs are kidney disease and Addison's disease. Depending upon the type and degree of the malfunction, their effects can be mild, causing few problems, or they can be life-threatening. In severe cases a pacemaker may be required for long-term management of the disorder.

Regardless of the underlying etiology, the symptoms associated with heart failure generally include coughing, especially at night and after exercise, breathing distress, weight loss, and exercise intolerance. Severely affected dogs may stand with their front legs spread wide apart and their neck lowered and extended to allow for easier passage of air into the lungs. Others may collapse after the slightest exertion or excitement. As mentioned previously, a distended abdomen may result when the right side of the heart is affected. In the case of left-sided heart failure, severe coughing and gagging with expectoration may occur.

Diagnosis of heart disease or failure begins with a thorough physical examination by your veterinarian. If disease involving the heart valves is present, heart murmurs are usually detectable upon chest auscultation with a stethoscope. Radiographs of the chest are almost always required for a definitive diagnosis of heart disease. Most diseased hearts appear abnormally enlarged on radiographic analysis. The enlargement occurs in compensation for the increased work load on the diseased heart or is due to thinning and bulging of the heart muscle.

In addition to the physical examination and radiographs, your veterinarian may order an electrocardiogram (ECG). A normal heartbeat is produced when a wave of electrical energy moves through the tissues of the heart chambers, starting at the top of the heart and moving down toward the apex. The electrical wave then causes the muscles lining those chambers to contract and expel the blood within. The purpose of the ECG is to evaluate the status of this electrical conduction system. With the information gained from this test, proper drug treatment dosages can be more easily established.

Since most cases of heart disease are nonreversible, the treatment goals for older dogs are first to reduce the work load on the diseased heart and then to slow the progression of the disease. Special diets that are low in sodium can be prescribed by veterinarians to help counteract the high blood pressure caused by the heart disease, thereby discouraging fluid build-up within the lungs or abdomen. In addition to special rations, diuretic medications such as furosemide are often prescribed to rid the body of excessive fluid that may be accumulating as a result of the malfunctioning heart. Keep in mind that diuretics cause a pet to drink more water and urinate more frequently than normal, at least until the body becomes accustomed to the medication. In more advanced disease, drugs designed to dilate the blood vessels and reduce the blood pressure even further may be required as well. Finally, if none of the above treatment regimens prove effective, a common final step is use of digitalis-derived medications to slow and strengthen the heart's contraction. Because those medicines can have many undesirable, serious side effects, older dogs taking them should be carefully monitored for abnormal signs.

Canine Heartworm Disease

Heartworm disease is a devastating, often fatal disease affecting dogs worldwide. It is caused by the organism *Dirofilaria immitis,* a worm that

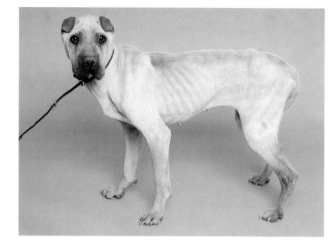

Cachexia associated with a severe case of canine heartworm disease.

normally lodges in the right chambers of the heart and in adjacent blood vessels. Adult heartworms are round and slender; they can reach 12 to 14 inches in length. In infected animals, they incite inflammation within the blood vessels and the lungs and can even obstruct circulation to other organs, including the liver and the kidneys. The worm burden in the heart and vessels can so greatly reduce the circulation of blood that unconsciousness or even sudden death results. In one case, over 200 worms were removed from the heart of a dog! Oftentimes the increased work load caused by the worms residing in the heart eventually weakens the heart muscle and leads to congestive heart failure. Left untreated, canine heartworm disease can ultimately take the life of the host.

Heartworm disease is transmitted from dog to dog by mosquitoes. When a mosquito feeds on an infected dog, heartworm larvae cir-

culating within the bloodstream (microfilariae) are ingested by the mosquito. While inside the mosquito, the larvae go through a two- to three-week development phase, during which time they become potentially infective to other dogs. Once maturation is complete, the infective larvae in the mosquito can enter the tissues of another dog when the mosquito feeds. After a short development period, the newly transplanted larvae begin to migrate through the tissues to the heart of their new host. This entire cycle, from initial transplantation to arrival at the heart, may take up to four months. Upon reaching the heart, the immature heartworms develop into sexually mature adults within two months. As adults, heartworms may reside within the heart and nearby blood vessels for many years, with female worms producing thousands of offspring and releasing them into the bloodstream. Once that happens, the larvae can be picked up by other mosquitoes and carried to dogs .

Clinical signs associated with heartworm disease in older dogs include lethargy, exercise intolerance, breathing difficulties, coughing, and a distended abdomen. Dogs infested with these parasites may go years without showing any clinical signs whatsoever; however, once signs do appear they are usually indicative of an advanced stage of the disease. Treatment at this time can be very difficult and unrewarding.

Heartworm disease can be diagnosed by a simple blood test. In the past detection of the microfilariae from blood samples drawn from dogs was the most reliable method of diagnosing canine heartworm disease. Now, however, recent technology has made the detection of these parasites easier and more reliable. New tests called enzyme immunoassays can detect the presence of adult worms within the heart and lungs and even estimate the number of worms there. This technology is important for several reasons. First, occult heartworm infections—infections characterized by the presence of adult heartworms with no circulating larvae—are not at all uncommon in dogs. The new tests can detect occult infections that might be missed by older testing methods, which target circulating larvae. Second, the new tests enable veterinarians to differentiate the canine heartworm, *Dirofilaria immitis,* from another type of worm that may be found in a dog's bloodstream, *Dipetalonema reconditum.* The latter organism is not considered dangerous to dogs, yet in the past its presence was often misdiagnosed as heartworms.

Heartworm disease usually can be treated, but the success of the treatment depends upon early detection of the disease and prompt initiation of therapy. The current compound used to treat heartworm disease in dogs is thiacetarsamide. This drug, administered intravenously, kills adult worms in the heart and lungs. Unfor-

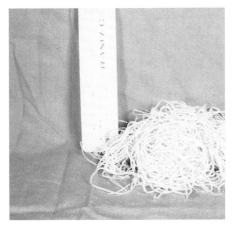

A cluster of heartworms removed from a single heart!

tunately, it is highly toxic and can damage the liver and kidneys of the dog being treated. This threat is especially significant in older dogs that may have existing impairment of these organs. In addition, although the medication kills most adult heartworms, some may escape its toxic effects, necessitating a repeat of treatment. Following treatment of adult heartworms, special medications are given to kill any remaining larvae in the bloodstream.

Fortunately, newer, safer drugs on the horizon show promise in treating this devastating disease. However, it is tragic that canine heartworm disease occurs at all, because it is so easily preventable. New safe, convenient preventive medications can be given once a month to protect dogs against these harmful parasites. Consult your veterinarian today if your pet is not currently taking heartworm preventive medication. It is easy to administer, safe, and well worth it! One word of caution: Heartworm preventive medication should never be given to your dog unless its blood has tested negative for heartworms. In a dog harboring heartworms, such medication can produce a severe, life-threatening reaction.

Anemia

The term anemia refers to a total reduction in the number of red blood cells circulating in the bloodstream. Anemia can be further classified as regenerative or nonregenerative, according to the body's ability to produce more red blood cells to replace those lost. Anemia results from one of three factors. The first of these, actual loss of red blood cells from the bloodstream, can be caused by internal or external hemorrhaging, parasites such as fleas, ticks, and hookworms, gastrointestinal ulcers such as those seen in older dogs with kidney failure, bleeding tumors, including hemangiosarcomas, blood clotting disorders, and urinary tract lesions. Second, anemia can result from an abnormal increase in the destruction of red blood cells within the body and bloodstream. The most common cause of that is autoimmune hemolytic anemia, a disease in which the dog's immune system attacks and destroys its own red blood cells because it mistakes them for foreign invaders. Severe bacterial and viral infections can also lead to increased destruction of red blood cells. Third, an overall decrease in the body's regular production of red blood cells can lead to or exacerbate an anemic state. Such a deficiency can occur secondarily to iron deficiencies (iron is needed for proper red blood cell production) caused in older dogs by poor diet or gastrointestinal disease. Other disorders that can cause an overall drop in red blood cell production include kidney disease, liver disease, hypothyroidism, Addison's disease, bone marrow disease, and long-term infection.

Anemia diminishes the amount of oxygen available for tissues and cells; as a result, clinical signs of oxygen deprivation are most apparent. Clinical signs associated with anemia include lethargy, weakness, labored breathing, and an overall pale or white appearance of the gums and other mucous membranes of the body. In addition, if red blood cells are being destroyed in the body, the mucous membranes may appear yellow owing to jaundice.

Anemia can be diagnosed through a laboratory blood analysis. Obviously, specific treatment depends

Check for anemia by examining the color of gums.

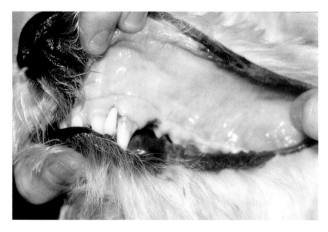

upon proper identification and treatment of the inciting condition. General treatments for this potentially life-threatening deficiency include blood transfusions, oxygen therapy, antibiotics, B-vitamins, and anabolic steroids. In cases of autoimmune hemolytic anemia, high doses of corticosteroids are needed to suppress the immune system and prevent further damage. Finally, high-quality, high-energy diets are usually prescribed to assist the body in replenishing its supply of red blood cells.

Bleeding Disorders

Hemostasis refers to the body's ability to control and stop bleeding that is occurring either inside or outside the body. Whenever a blood vessel is torn or damaged by trauma or disease, a chain reaction begins in the body to stop the escape of blood from the perforated vessel. The first event in this sequence is the constriction of the damaged vessel to slow the blood loss. Upon constriction, special cells within the blood called platelets begin adhering to the vessel wall at the site of injury and form a plug to contain the blood within the vessel. At the same time the coagulation pathway is activated. That involves a complex interaction of blood cells and blood components, as well as calcium and vitamin K. The primary purpose of the coagulation pathway is to reinforce, strengthen, and stabilize the clot formed by the platelets.

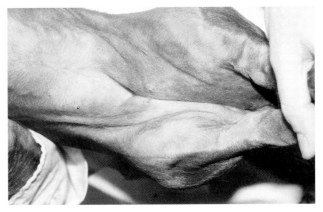

Disruption of this hemostatic chain of events along any part of the pathway can lead to uncontrolled bleeding in a pet. For instance, the diseases and agents that cause thrombocytopenia, or a decrease of the total number of platelets in the blood, can cause bleeding disorders. Agents that can induce thrombocytopenia include bacterial toxins, bacterial agents (ehrlichiosis), autoimmune diseases, drugs used for cancer therapy, and diseases that affect the bone marrow. In addition, whenever a dog experiences a serious disease or injury, a condition known as disseminated intravascular coagulation (DIC) can occur. DIC, characterized by the formation of small blood clots throughout the body, causes an overall depletion of platelets and other clotting components. Continued depletion can leave the body vulnerable to unchecked hemorrhage, which can kill if the DIC is not brought under control.

Instead of actually causing thrombocytopenia, certain medical

Bruising associated with a bleeding disorder.

conditions simply interfere with the normal function of platelets and predispose an older dog to bleeding. Such conditions include liver disease, kidney disease, and neoplasia of various types. In addition, select medications that may be used in older dogs can have an adverse effect on platelet function. Aspirin, often prescribed for arthritis in older dogs, is one such medication. Omega-3 fatty acids, used to treat allergies in dogs, can have the same effect in exceptionally high doses.

Aside from actual alterations in platelet numbers and function, bleeding disorders can be caused by deficiencies in calcium and in vitamin K. The latter type is often seen in dogs that have ingested rat poison. Finally, any interference with or deficiencies in the clotting factors involved in the coagulation pathway, as with the disease hemophilia, also predispose a pet to uncontrolled bleeding. Liver disease is also known to cause bleeding disorders in older dogs, because many of the components in the hemostatic pathway are manufactured in the liver.

Symptoms seen in pets with dysfunctions in the hemostatic pathway include bruising and subcutaneous hemorrhaging affecting the skin and mucous membranes. Often, blood may be evident in a dog's urine and fecal material. Spontaneous nosebleeds have been known to occur, as well as joint swelling, pain, and subsequent lameness as blood fills the joint spaces. Last, loss of blood from

poor hemostasis, often produces signs of anemia as well.

Because of the wide variety of potential etiologies for bleeding disorders, a series of laboratory tests will be required to pinpoint the cause of a dog's bleeding tendencies. Once that is determined, a correct treatment regimen can be started. It may include, aside from other specific treatments, blood transfusions, vitamin K injections (if rodenticide poisoning is suspected), and corticosteroid therapy if autoimmune disease is present.

The Respiratory System

The function of the respiratory system is to provide oxygen to, and remove carbon dioxide from, the circulatory system. Since oxygen is required for all metabolic reactions within the body, unimpeded functioning of this system is vital to the continuance of life processes. In dogs the respiratory system also serves as the primary method of thermoregulation for the body, by transferring heat with each exhaled breath. Remember: Our canine friends don't sweat when they get hot, they pant. The respiratory system begins with the nose and mouth. Next comes the trachea, a tubular structure composed of firm, cartilaginous support rings that maintain its cylindrical shape. After entering the chest cavity, the trachea splits into two bronchi, which branch even further into smaller units. The alveoli, which are formed by the lung tissue, are fed by those units. It is in the alveoli that oxygen and carbon dioxide are exchanged between the lungs and the circulatory system.

Tracheobronchitis

Tracheobronchitis is inflammation affecting the trachea and bronchi. In older dogs the primary cause of this type of inflammation is canine cough complex. Canine cough is a disease that can be caused by a number of different organisms, including the parainfluenza virus, the canine adenovirus, and the *Bordetella* bacterium. Highly contagious, it is characterized by a dry hacking cough that appears one to two weeks after exposure. It can be especially hard on older dogs with weakened immune systems. If it is left untreated, the organisms responsible can damage the lining of the trachea and bronchi. That leads to permanent scarring and increased susceptibility to secondary infections. Fortunately, keeping older dogs current on vaccinations greatly diminishes the likelihood of contracting canine cough.

Noninfectious causes of tracheobronchitis include foreign matter, allergies, or other irritants that have entered the airways. As with canine cough, incessant coughing is the primary clinical sign. These coughs may be moist and productive, rather than dry and hacking, however.

Tracheobronchitis is diagnosed by means of clinical signs, history of recent exposure to other dogs, physical exam findings, and, if necessary, radiographs of the trachea and lungs. Treatment of tracheobronchitis consists of antibiotic therapy when appropriate. In cases that prove refractory to antimicrobial therapy, cultures of the respiratory secretions may be needed to determine the type of organism involved. In cases with dry, unproductive coughing, cough-suppressant medication may be used as well. Such medications should not be used if the cough is moist and productive, however, since they interfere with the body's natural ability to rid the lungs and airways of undesirable substances. In these instances, vaporizers can help liquify the secretions in the airway to allow greater ease of passage. If a foreign object or tumor is causing the airway inflammation, removal by surgery or endoscopy is warranted.

Collapsed Trachea

Tracheal collapse is a condition caused by a weakening of the muscles that support the rings of cartilage lining the trachea. When that occurs, the trachea becomes prone to collapse during normal respiration, with resultant oxygen deprivation. Small, toy breeds of dogs over six years of age are the most likely candidates for this disorder.

Dogs suffering from tracheal collapse exhibit signs of respiratory distress, including a wide-based stance, neck extension, and open-mouth breathing. A characteristic

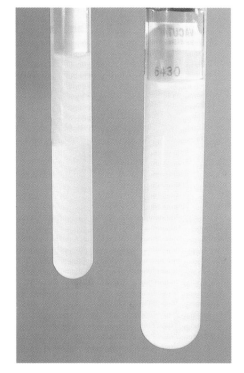

dry, harsh cough like the honk of a goose is heard as well.

Diagnosis of tracheal collapse is dependent upon physical exam findings and radiographs of the throat region. In addition, examination of the trachea with an endoscope is diagnostic and can pinpoint the site of the collapse.

Depending upon the severity of the clinical signs, a collapsed trachea can be managed either medically or surgically. Mild cases often can be managed through the use of cough suppressants and drugs that dilate the airways to compensate for the collapse. To prevent overexertion, supervision of activity is also warranted. In more severe cases,

surgical correction, involving implantation of artificial support rings, can afford a cure.

Pneumothorax, Pulmonary Edema, and Pleural Effusions

Pneumothorax is a life-threatening condition caused by the influx of air into the chest cavity, either through a wound penetrating into the chest, or through tissue damage in the bronchi or lungs caused by trauma or by an invasive tumor. The resulting loss of the negative pressure that normally exists within the chest cavity can collapse the lungs and lead to profound respiratory distress. If negative pressure is not restored quickly, either through the use of air drainage tubes or by surgical repair of the hole or tear, death can be swift.

The accumulation of fluid or discharge, rather than air, within the chest cavity is referred to as pleural effusion. These effusions, which usually consist primarily of blood, pus, or lymph, can put great pressure on the lungs and cause respiratory distress. One such effusion, hemothorax, or the presence of blood in the chest cavity, is attributable to trauma, blood clotting disorders, heartworms, or disorders of the blood vessels supplying the lungs. Pyothorax, the accumulation of pus in this cavity, is due to infection of the lungs or pleural space with pus-forming bacteria. Chylothorax, the build-up of lymph in the chest cavity, commonly occurs secondary to tumors or inflammation involving the lymphatic chain and located in the chest cavity.

Effusions are accumulations of fluid within the chest cavity; pulmonary edema is the accumulation of fluid within the lung tissue itself. Here respiratory distress is caused by lack of oxygen exchange rather than by abnormal amounts of pressure on the lungs. The causes of pulmonary edema in older dogs include congestive heart failure, electric shock, and allergic reactions. Other less-common causes are aspiration of stomach contents into the lungs and inhalation of toxic fumes.

Dogs with pleural effusions or pulmonary edema exhibit breathing difficulties and show intense lethargy, exercise intolerance, and the peculiar stances or postures associated with respiratory distress. A definitive diagnosis of an effusion can be achieved by means of a radiograph of the chest or through the use of a fine needle aspirate and microscopic examination of the fluid contents.

Pulmonary edema is treated by first addressing the underlying cause and then, if necessary utilizing special drugs designed to move the fluid out of the lungs. Pleural effusions are treated by removing the fluid from the chest cavity with a needle and syringe or, in severe cases, by installing a temporary drainage tube in the chest. Once the immediate distress has been relieved, a search for the underlying cause of the effusion can be sought. That is important, since identification and treatment of the underlying cause is the only way to afford a complete cure and to prevent recurrence.

Pneumonia

Pneumonia arises when inflammation or infection strikes the lungs. It is especially serious in older dogs, which may already be suffering from oxygen deprivation due to heart disease or age-related degeneration of lung capacity. Causes of pneumonia in older dogs are numerous. Secondary bacterial pneumonias are not uncommon in dogs whose immune systems have been stressed by other illnesses, such as kidney failure. Fungal diseases such as blastomycosis, histoplasmosis, and coccidioidomycosis can stimulate granuloma formation in the lungs and create a severe pneumonia. Aspiration pneumonia, caused by accidental inhalation of food or liquid, can appear in older dogs with oral or esophageal disease or in canines suffering from seizures or persistent vomiting. Lung inflammation can also result from inhalation of smoke and certain caustic chemicals. Finally, fluid build-up within the lungs caused by heart disease or neoplasia, and encroachment upon healthy lung tissue by tumor growth can also result in a pneumonic state.

Clinical signs of pneumonia include persistent coughing, fever, lethargy, and inappetence. A wide-based stance with neck extended

Pneumonia.

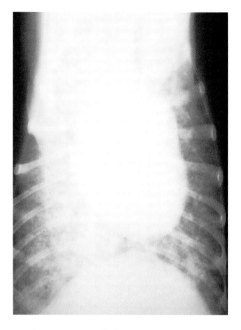

and open-mouth breathing may also be seen. Of course, the degree of breathing difficulty is determined by the amount of lung tissue affected.

Definitive diagnosis of pneumonia and its underlying cause can be made through stethoscopic evaluation of the lungs at work and through radiographs of the lung fields. In addition, blood profiles may be run to determine whether an infectious component is present. If a bacterial or fungal infection is suspected, a culture of respiratory fluid and discharge may be taken to identify the causative organism and to select an appropriate treatment.

Treatment of pneumonia usually consists of antibiotic or antifungal therapy to treat any infection present or to prevent the appearance of a secondary infection, drug therapy

designed to move fluid out of the lungs and expand the airways for increased oxygen flow into the lungs, and, in select cases, medications aimed at reducing inflammation in the lungs. Intravenous fluids are also prescribed for patients with advanced cases of pneumonia, to help replace body fluids lost through increased respiratory secretions and to prevent existing secretions from becoming thickened as a result of dehydration. As a rule, medications designed to suppress coughing are not used in dogs with pneumonia, since they would only slow the expulsion of mucus and other excess secretions from the lungs. Stress reduction and forced rest are essential if recovery is to occur.

Chronic Obstructive Pulmonary Disease (COPD)

Chronic obstructive pulmonary disease is a disorder of the lungs and respiratory tree often linked to aging in dogs. COPD is actually a catch-all term for conditions that affect and restrict normal air movement into and within the lungs. Chronic bronchitis and age-related scarring of the lung tissue are the most common causes of COPD in senior canines.

COPD is characterized by persistent coughing, mucus buildup within the airways, and breathing difficulties. Definitive diagnosis of chronic obstructive pulmonary disease can be made by ruling out other potential causes of the clinical signs (such as pneumonia and canine cough), evaluating the duration of the clinical signs, and obtaining biopsy samples of lung tissue to determine scar tissue is present. Unfortunately, there is no treatment that can reverse the effects of COPD. However, medications (such as theophylline and aminophylline) designed to dilate the airway passages can provide some degree of respiratory relief. In addition, anti-inflammatory medications can be utilized to reduce inflammation and slow scar tissue formation that may be contributing to the COPD.

The Urinary System

The urinary system removes metabolic waste material from the bloodstream and regulates fluid balance within the body. It consists of two kidneys, which are responsible for filtering wastes out of the blood, and ureters, which transport urine from the kidneys to the bladder, where the urine is stored until voided from the body via the urethra. Another important function of the kidneys is to assist in the production of a special hormone, called erythropoietin, which stimulates the production of red blood cells in the body and indirectly regulates blood pressure.

Kidney Disease and Kidney Failure

Kidney disease is one of the most common disorders associated with aging in canines. As kidney tissues

deteriorate with age through normal wear and tear and scar tissue replaces healthy tissue, the kidneys decrease in size and slowly lose their ability to filter wastes out of the blood with efficiency. As the scarring and loss of healthy cells within the kidneys progress, those organs will gradually fail; toxins and waste material will steadily build up within the body and produce clinical signs and severe consequences.

Factors that can further damage kidney cells and expedite kidney degeneration and failure in older dogs include poisons such as ethylene glycol (antifreeze), trauma, heart disease, and autoimmune diseases. In addition, certain medications, when used for prolonged periods or in exceptionally high doses, can damage the kidneys. Examples of such medications are aspirin and certain antibiotics. Finally, bacterial infections originating in periodontal disease, pyometras, prostate infections, or bladder infections can contribute significantly to kidney disease in older dogs.

The symptoms associated with kidney disease can be quite variable, depending on the extent of the damage. In fact, symptoms will not even be apparent until over 70 percent of total kidney function has been lost. When symptoms do arise, the more quickly therapeutic measures are undertaken the more favorable the response to treatment will be. Kidney failure presents itself in two basic forms. The first presentation, acute kidney failure, is characterized

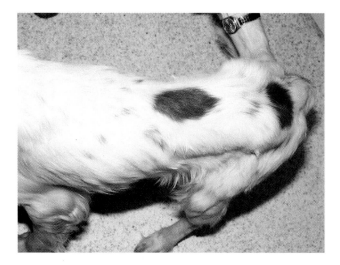

Muscle atrophy and wasting associated with kidney disease.

term progression of illness and clinical signs. Dogs suffering from chronic kidney failure exhibit depression, loss of appetite, increased thirst, and increased desire to urinate (see Urination, Excessive, p. 152). Slow buildups of waste products in the bloodstream can also promote the formation of ulcers in the stomach or elsewhere in the gastrointestinal tract and lend an ammonia scent to the breath of affected dogs. Finally, dogs suffering from chronic kidney failure can experience anemia, since the kidney plays an important role in the production of red blood cells.

Diagnosis of kidney disease can be made through a series of laboratory tests performed on the blood and urine. By evaluating blood urea nitrogen (BUN) and creatinine levels within the blood and comparing them with the specific gravity of the urine, veterinarians are able to make a preliminary determination concerning kidney status. If a problem is suspected, hospitalization for further testing may be required to determine the extent of the functional compromise.

Left untreated, chronic kidney disease can lead directly to an acute crisis. Unfortunately, kidney dialysis for dogs is currently not a practical treatment alternative, because of prohibitive costs and the lack of patient cooperation. If other therapeutic measures are instituted quickly enough and with consistency, however, chronic kidney failure can be a manageable

by intense dehydration, vomiting, shock, unconsciousness, and often sudden death. Nearly all kidney function has been lost, and the body has no effective means of ridding itself of waste. The most frequent causes of sudden failure include ingestion of antifreeze, direct trauma to the kidneys causing extensive structural damage, and overwhelming infections. In addition, urinary tract obstructions such as those seen in urolithiasis, can lead to kidney damage by causing a backflow of urine and a subsequent increase in pressure within the kidneys. Dogs experiencing acute kidney failure must be treated vigorously with intravenous fluids to correct water and electrolyte imbalances, and with medications designed to stimulate kidney function. If treatment is instituted soon enough, acute kidney failure often can be reversed.

In contrast, chronic kidney failure is characterized by a slower, longer-

condition. Although the degenerative changes cannot be reversed, their progression can often be slowed through proper treatment.

First, provide unlimited access to clean, fresh water to dogs with kidney disease, to satisfy increases in thirst and effectively stimulate their kidneys. Depriving a dog with chronic renal failure of water for even a short time could induce an acute crisis. Second, special diets available from veterinarians should replace existing rations. These diets, by reducing the amount of waste material produced during the digestive process, help to keep toxins at the lowest level possible (see Nutrition for Your Older Dog, p. 9). Third, drugs to help regulate calcium and phosphorus levels within the body, antiulcer medications to counteract the toxic effects on the lining of the gastrointestinal tract, and diuretic medications, such as furosemide, that stimulate the kidneys to increase urine output may all be prescribed to alleviate clinical signs. Finally, a key to the management of chronic kidney disease is to address any underlying sources that may be contributing to the problem. For instance, conditions such as periodontal disease must be addressed at the same time, to prevent continued deterioration. Pet owners must also be aware that even mild episodes of vomiting or diarrhea can have profound effects on the water and pH balance in the body of older dogs with kidney compromise. Rapid dehydration and associated complications can result. Seek prompt veterinary attention if these symptoms arise.

Urinary Tract Infections

Infections of the urinary system can have their origin in any portion of the urinary tract, or they can occur secondarily to infections of the reproductive organs, such as the uterus or prostate gland. In healthy dogs, special defense mechanisms within the urinary system prevent an infection from gaining a foothold. For instance, antibodies lining the surface of the bladder and urethra provide an initial line of defense against bacteria. Further, sphincters consisting of thick bands of muscle are situated in strategic areas along the urinary tract to help seal off portions of the tract from one another and to limit the spread of infection. The pH of the urine is another safeguard against infection. The acidic urine normally produced by dogs is generally inhibitory to the growth of bacteria. Finally, frequent, consistent urination is an important means of eliminating bacteria that may have penetrated the lower portions of the urinary system. Any disruption of the normal routine of urination can predispose a dog to a urinary tract infection.

Certainly the vast majority of urinary tract infections are caused by bacteria that gain entrance to the body through the external opening of the urethra and evade the normal defense mechanisms, which may

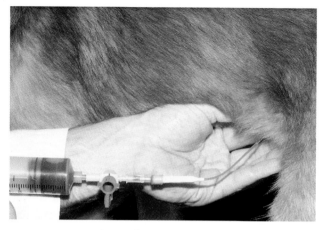

Collecting urine for laboratory analysis. Note the dark color of the urine, caused by infection.

Straining to urinate, bloody urine, continual licking at the urethral opening, and increased water consumption are symptoms of urinary tract infection. In severe cases, fever, depression, and inappetence may accompany those signs. However, many dogs with urinary tract infection show no clinical signs whatsoever. In these instances, infections often remain unnoticed until detected in a routine laboratory examination.

Prompt diagnosis and treatment of urinary tract infections are essential to ensure complete elimination of the infection and to prevent its spread into vital areas of the kidneys. Diagnosis of a urinary tract infection is accomplished through the use of clinical signs, urine evaluations, and, if deemed necessary, urine cultures to identify specific bacteria. Blood tests can also rule out underlying causes such as diabetes mellitus and Cushing's disease. If urinary stones, anatomical defects, or tumors are suspected, radiographs will be taken as well.

Treatment of urinary tract infections involves the administration of specific antibiotics for 10 days to two weeks. In older dogs suffering from chronic bouts of infection, a maintenance dose of antibiotics once daily may be prescribed to keep the bacteria growth under control. The dose is usually given just before bedtime to allow high concentrations to build up within the urine overnight.

Other preventive measures include providing plenty of fresh

have been weakened by stress or a nonrelated disease. Female dogs are more prone to infection in this manner because their urethral passage, much shorter than that of males, allows for easier passage of bacteria. In other cases, infectious organisms can travel through the blood, lymphatic system, or penetrating wounds and infect the various organs of the urinary system. Other disease processes too can predispose a dog to urinary tract infections. For example, a high sugar content in the urine of a dog suffering from diabetes creates a prime growth medium for bacteria. In addition, diseases causing nerve damage or sphincter damage to the bladder and urethra can weaken the body's defense mechanisms and lead to a secondary infection. Further, anatomical defects caused by injury, uroliths (stones), and tumors can act as a nidus for infection. Consequently, if infections are recurring, a search for an underlying cause should be made.

drinking water and allowing frequent trips outdoors to eliminate. Special diets also help by regulating the pH of the urine, thereby affecting bacterial growth. Finally, in female dogs, keeping the hair coat surrounding the vulva trimmed short will discourage bacteria contaminating the hair from ascending up the urethra and into the bladder.

Urolithiasis (Urinary Stones)

Urinary tract infections that are not treated in a timely manner can result in urolithiasis, or stone formation within the urinary system. Bacteria within the urine begin to break down some of the urine components and alter the pH of the urine. When this alteration occurs, special crystals called struvite can form within the urine, and they in turn can coalesce into actual stones within the bladder. Not all uroliths are caused by bacterial infection, though. Some stones result from inherent metabolic disorders, and in these instances, cystine or urate crystals are the usual precursors, rather than struvite crystals.

In general, female dogs are more prone to struvite crystal formation

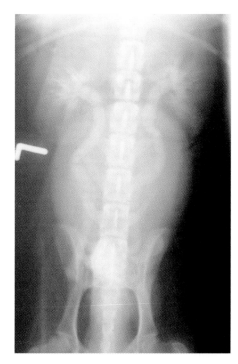

Grossly distended bladder and ureters caused by a urinary obstruction.

than are males, primarily because they are more prone to bladder infections. However, urinary stones can be especially dangerous in male dogs if they become lodged within the urethra and are unable to pass. If they are not dislodged in a timely manner, obstruction of urine flow can result in kidney damage.

Symptoms associated with urolithiasis are similar to those of urinary tract infection. Affected dogs exhibit pronounced stranguria (straining to urinate), which may or may not produce urine from the urethral opening. Interestingly, however, some dogs, especially females, show no clinical signs, yet have a bladder full of stones. These cases are often discovered acciden-

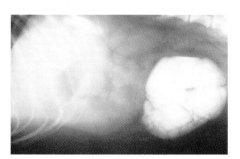

Uroliths filling a bladder.

67

tally, when routine abdominal radiographs are taken as part of a geriatric preventive health care screen.

Diagnosis of urinary stones is based upon urinalysis findings, rectal palpation of the bladder, and, in some cases, radiographs. Not all uroliths show up on radiographs. Stones composed of urate or cystine crystals require special contrast radiographs for identification. In male dogs, if blockage is suspected, passage of a urinary catheter will be performed to dislodge any stones in an effort to reestablish urine flow.

When no obstruction is present, urolith removal is accomplished by either dietary or surgical means, depending upon size. Smaller uroliths and crystals can usually be effectively dissolved with specially modified diets designed for that purpose. This type of therapy may continue for four months before a cure is achieved. Stones that are too large to dissolve by dietary means may need to be shattered ultrasonically or surgically removed. If an infection is suspected to be the underlying cause of the urolithiasis, antibiotic therapy is indicated as well. Once the crystals and stones have been eliminated, special diets will be prescribed to discourage reformation.

The Reproductive System

The reproductive system can become a significant source of medical challenges in mature dogs that have not been neutered. Reproductive efficiency begins its decline in dogs after eight years of age. Influenced over the years by unique and prolonged hormonal patterns, the reproductive tissues of these dogs can experience abnormal anatomical growth or secretory activity. The changes, if significant, can predispose the pet to a number of serious medical conditions.

The reproductive system of the female canine consists of the ovaries (which produce eggs and reproductive hormones), the oviducts (where fertilization takes place), the uterus (the site of fetal development), the birth canal, and the mammary glands. In older intact females, the sites of most troubles are the uterus and the mammary glands (see Cancer in Older Dogs, p. 114). Of the various male reproductive organs, which include the testicles and associated structures, the penis, and the prostate gland, it is the prostate that seems to cause the most problems as aging occurs. As a general rule, neutering at a young age can minimize these challenges.

Metritis and Cystic Endometrial Hyperplasia Complex (Pyometra)

Unspayed female dogs over the age of six are very susceptible to metritis and cystic endometrial hyperplasia complex (CEHC), also known as pyometra. Metritis is inflammation involving the lining of the uterus; CEHC is a condition in which the uterus becomes distended with uterine secretions and inflammatory fluid.

The causes of metritis are numerous. They can include venereal disease organisms, endocrine disorders such as diabetes mellitus, abnormal pregnancies or births, and treatments with certain types of drugs, especially hormones used to prevent or terminate unwanted pregnancies. Pyometra has its origins in the reproductive hormonal cycles that occur year after year. Growth of the glands within the inner walls of the uterus is promoted by high levels of the hormone progesterone, which is secreted by the ovaries toward the end of a dog's heat cycle. Progesterone increases fluid secretions from these glands and decreases uterine muscle motility. These conditions ultimately lead to fluid accumulation within the uterus. The fluid may escape from the uterus in the form of a discharge. However, if for some reason it is not allowed to escape, a dangerous pyometra can result, with marked uterine enlargement, even to the point of rupture. Further, since the retained fluid is an ideal medium for the growth of bacteria and other organisms, infection can arise. In advanced cases the bacteria and the toxins they produce can enter the bloodstream and cause blood poisoning. In addition, kidney failure can occur secondary to pyometra, because of the immune response mounted by the body to combat the infection.

The most prevalent clinical sign of metritis is a thick yellow-green to hemorrhagic vaginal discharge. In addition, constant grooming around the vaginal opening is common in dogs with metritis. In advanced cases, loss of appetite, fever, and abdominal pain may occur as well. Finally, owing to the close proximity of the urinary and reproductive systems in female dogs, secondary bladder infections can arise.

Dogs with pyometra exhibit signs similar to those of metritis, though a discharge is not necessarily present. Moreover, true pyometra classically causes a marked increase in thirst and abdominal enlargement. If secondary kidney disease becomes a factor, dehydration, vomiting, or increased urination may occur as well.

Diagnosis of metritis and pyometra is made on the basis of a history (indicating, for example, whether the dog is intact or neutered), clinical signs, and a laboratory workup including blood tests, discharge cultures, or abdominal radiographs. In cases of pyometra, blood work often reveals a marked elevation of the white blood cell count and a mild anemic state. Abdominal radiographs reveal a grossly distended uterus that displaces other organs within the abdomen.

The treatment of choice for both diseases is neutering. Although select cases of metritis may be treated successfully with antibiotic and fluid therapy, the chance of recurrence is so high that neutering should still be considered. In addition, even though special medications such as prostaglandin F2 alpha are sometimes used to treat pyometra in valuable breeding females, they should not be used for that purpose in dogs over eight years of age. Pyometra in an older dog is an emergency situation, and surgical removal of the uterus should be performed as soon as possible.

Prostate Disorders

As non-neutered male dogs increase in years, their susceptibility to prostate malfunctions also increases. Disorders that often affect the prostate of an older dog include bacterial infections, enlargements (benign prostatic hypertrophy), cysts, and tumors. General signs associated with prostate disease are straining to urinate, painful urination, blood in the urine, fever, abdominal pain, and thin ribbon-like stools (due to compression of the colon by the enlarged prostate). Hind limb lameness and edema, or water retention, in the hind limbs can occur if prostate enlargement impedes lymphatic drainage from the legs. In addition, prostate infections can be the source of recurring urinary tract infections and associated signs in male dogs.

Confirmation of prostate disease in older dogs is obtained by physical examination, radiography, or ultrasonography. If neoplasia is suspected, radiographs of the chest may also be taken to determine whether the cancer has spread to the lungs. In addition, fluid may be drained from the prostate with a catheter and examined microscopically for tumor cells or used to obtain bacterial cultures. Prostate cytology may be obtained by inserting a fine needle into the organ and withdrawing cells and tissue for microscopic examination.

Treatment of prostate disorders is dependent upon the underlying cause. For instance, prostate infections are treated with antibiotics or surgical drainage or both, depending upon the extent of the infection. When tumors or cysts are present, however, surgical intervention is usually required. Finally, neutering is recommended for all dogs suffering from benign prostatic hypertrophy or any other type of prostate disease.

The Musculoskeletal System

The musculoskeletal system of dogs, consisting of bones, muscles, joints, and the associated structures, provides locomotory ability and protects and supports vital internal organs. Accordingly, this system is designed to withstand the enormous amounts of wear and tear that accompany those important duties. Like other organ systems, however, it is not immune to the effects of aging, which are reflected in a number of musculoskeletal disease conditions prevalent in the aging dog population.

Arthritis and Osteoarthrosis

Arthritis is defined as inflammation involving one or more joints of the body, with or without accompanying bony changes in the joints in question. It usually manifests itself as lameness and swollen, painful joints. In older dogs, arthritis is most often caused by abnormal stress on a joint due to a previous injury or due to anatomical anomalies that may have been present since birth. For example, patellar luxation, a disease caused by anatomical deficiencies involving the knee joint, over time can produce serious arthritic changes in the knees of affected dogs. Additionally, arthritis can be caused by infectious organisms that have invaded a joint or by an overactive immune system that is attacking joint tissue (immune-mediated arthritis). In the last two instances, fever, loss of appetite, and general malaise usually accompany the arthritic symptoms.

Diagnosis of arthritis is made through the use of clinical signs, physical exam findings, and radiographs of the joints. If an infection is suspected, testing and evaluation of fluid obtained from an affected joint will be performed to identify the causative organism and to determine which medications will afford the quickest results. As far as immune-mediated arthritis is concerned, the two most prevalent types in geriatric canines are rheumatoid arthritis and SLE (systemic lupus erythematosus). Diagnosis and differentiation of these conditions can be definitively achieved with special blood tests and with biopsy samples of tissue and fluid from affected joints.

Treatment of arthritis that is non-infectious in nature employs anti-inflammatory medications, the strength of which is dependent upon the severity of the condition. Mild, early cases often can be managed with aspirin alone; advanced cases may require the use of steroid anti-inflammatories, as well as special drugs such as PSGAG (see p. 72). If an immune-mediated arthritis is diagnosed, even higher dosages of steroid anti-inflammatories will be required for management. Finally, treatment for infectious arthritis entails the use of appropriate antibiotics and antimicrobial medications, as well as surgical drainage and flushes of the affected joints in select instances.

Osteoarthrosis, or degenerative joint disease, has its origins in abnormal anatomy and biomechanics of one or more joints. Such abnormalities may be caused by trauma or by normal, age-related wear and tear to the joint, or they may be genetically induced. Canine hip dysplasia is probably the most notorious form of osteoarthrosis that is genetic in origin. Because of the variation in joint shape and function, the excessive wear and tear of the joint ligaments and the cartilages lining the joint surfaces leads to surface erosions. When that happens, the bony surfaces within the joint are allowed to rub against one another. Sharp pain and weakness are the results. Further, the rubbing action causes more surface changes, and a vicious cycle of disease is created. Affected dogs have difficulty in arising from recumbency, and they experience initial stiffness and lameness when in motion. The pain can cause behavior changes, including increased irritability. In addition, as activity levels decline because of the osteoarthrosis, atrophy of the muscles surrounding the joint(s) generally ensues.

Diagnosis of osteoarthrosis is based on radiographs of suspected joints and on the presence of this disorder in the dog's genetic bloodline. Treatment for the condition consists of moderate daily exercise to strengthen the muscles and tendons underlying and supporting the affected joint. Anti-inflammatory medications are used to relieve pain. In severe cases of osteoarthrosis, surgical intervention may be required to debride and rebuild the joints in an attempt to restore relatively pain-free function. Promising results also have been obtained with the drug polysulfated glycosaminoglycan (PSGAG) in dogs ravaged by hip dysplasia. PSGAG, by stimulating and encouraging the repair of damaged joint cartilage, effectively relieves the pain associated with bone-to-bone contact.

Spondylosis Deformans

Spondylosis deformans is a degenerative bone disease often seen in older, larger, more active breeds of dogs. Its exact cause remains a mystery, although certain aging changes affecting bone metabolism and calcium distribution are suspect. The hallmark of the disease is the development of bony outgrowths from the disks and vertebrae along the spinal column. The lumbar area of the spine, located between the rib cage and the pelvis, is the site usually involved. Dogs afflicted with this condition may show no clinical signs for years; however, as the condition progresses the bony outgrowths can cause pressure on the nerves leaving the spinal cord and pain in the surrounding musculature. That results in noticeable hind limb weakness and a reluctance to move. In severe instances the entire hind end becomes nonfunctional.

Definitive diagnosis of spondylosis deformans is achieved through radiographic analysis of the spinal column. These radiographs are important, since without them, dogs suffering from this condition might be misdiagnosed as having arthritic hips. Unfortunately, there is no cure for spondylosis deformans. Affected dogs are usually treated with anti-inflammatory medications such as aspirin and dexamethasone to reduce associated pain and inflammation. Anabolic steroids may also be used to help rebuild musculature in the hips and rear legs.

Knee Injuries

As muscle mass and ligament flexibility are lost with advancing years or with chronic disease, older dogs become more susceptible to knee injuries, specifically to torn cruciate ligaments. The knee joint is held together by a tough joint capsule made up of fibrous tissue and numerous ligaments, the most prominent of which are the cruciate ligaments. If abnormal force or exertion is placed upon the aged and weakened joint, one or more of the ligaments may rupture. Obesity can also place a great strain on these ligaments over time and predispose them to tears. Regardless of the cause, the joint instability that follows such injuries will eventually lead to arthritic changes within the joint itself if the condition is not treated.

Acute cruciate tears usually result in a sudden non-weight-bearing lameness. Within two to four days, function usually returns to the affected limb; however, a limp will be evident. Further, the limp tends to worsen with activity or as arthritis strikes the affected joint.

Diagnosis of a torn cruciate ligament is made by physical examination and evaluation of knee stability upon manipulation. Radiographs may be helpful in determining the duration and the extent of the injury as well. Upon diagnosis, the choice of the treatment mode will depend upon the severity of the injury and upon the weight and overall condition of the patient. In general,

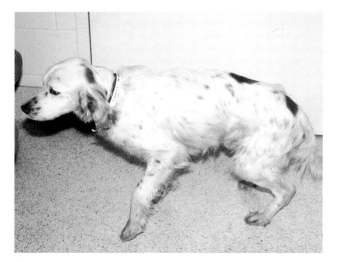

larger, more active dogs with severe tears require surgical joint restoration in order to regain stability and function. Smaller dogs that are at their proper body weight, however, may regain acceptable joint stability and function through the body's normal repair mechanisms. However, the risk of arthritic changes in these joints over time is still high if surgery is not performed.

Hindlimb weakness such as this can be caused by spondylosis deformans.

Metabolic Bone Disease

Older dogs suffering from kidney disease are susceptible to a metabolic condition known as secondary hyperparathyroidism, which is characterized by a generalized degeneration and thinning of bone. Elevated levels of phosphorus in the bloodstream caused by poor kidney function stimulate the body to draw calcium out of bony tissue in order to counter the phosphorus rise with a rise in blood calcium. Unfortunately, the effect on bone integrity can be

Knee joint instability will result from torn cruciate ligaments.

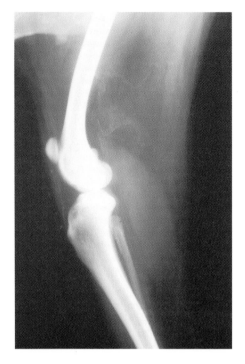

devastating. Dogs with metabolic bone disease experience lameness, weakness, joint deformities, and oftentimes spontaneous fractures as a result of this response.

Diagnosis of secondary hyperparathyroidism is based upon a diagnosis of kidney disease and upon the detection of elevated calcium levels in the blood. In addition, radiographic skeletal findings can be used to confirm the diagnosis. Treatment of the disease includes management of the underlying kidney disease and, in some cases, administration of calcium supplements. Unfortunately, since many cases of kidney disease in older dogs are progressive, a complete cure is unlikely.

Myositis/Myopathy

When inflammation strikes the muscle tissue of older dogs, the term myositis is used. Myositis results in weakness and atrophy in the muscle groups affected. Affected dogs are reluctant to move because of the pain involved. In addition, when touched, they may vocalize or exhibit aggressive behavior.

The causes of myositis in older dogs can include trauma, infection, autoimmune disease, and poor circulation secondary to heart disease. Diagnosis of the underlying cause is based upon clinical signs and laboratory blood tests designed to detect elevations in muscle enzymes and white blood cells. In those cases in which myositis is suspected yet the blood work remains inconclusive, a biopsy of affected muscle tissue is indicated as well. A cure, of course, depends upon identification and treatment of the underlying cause. Antibiotics are used if an infection is present, and, in most cases, anti-inflammatory drugs can reduce the pain and discomfort originating from the muscles. Myositis induced by an overactive immune system is treated with high doses of glucocorticosteroids or similar medications designed to suppress the inflated immune response. Finally, if poor circulation is to blame, concurrent treatment with drugs designed to improve blood flow to the muscles is appropriate.

Myopathy is the actual degeneration of muscle cells and tissue structure. It results in pronounced muscle atrophy, weakness, and gait abnormalities. Even eating, drinking, and breathing may be affected as the muscles responsible for those functions experience degeneration as well. Unlike myositis, a myopathic condition is not necessarily accompanied by pain.

Unfortunately for pets suffering from a degenerative myopathy, there is no specific treatment that can stop or reverse the course of the disease. Symptomatic treatment with anti-inflammatory medications may provide temporary relief from pain and discomfort.

Perineal Hernia

Perineal hernias result from a weakening of the muscles just beneath the tail on either side of the anal opening. Seen primarily in old, intact male dogs, these hernias present as abnormal bulgings or swellings caused by intestinal protrusion through the muscle wall. They are normally soft and fluctuant to the touch. Because a perineal hernia impairs the ability to defecate and often traps fecal material within its pouch, affected dogs often exhibit straining upon defecation and other signs of constipation.

Diagnosis of this condition can usually be made upon physical examination. In addition, radiographs are useful in determining the extent of fecal impaction caused by the herniation. Treatment involves manual evacuation of the colon and hernia pocket of fecal material with warm-water enemas.

Once that is accomplished, surgical correction of the hernia can be performed. Afterward, the dogs are placed on high-fiber diets to facilitate normal evacuation of the colon and to reduce the pressure placed on the perineal region by the act of defecation. One important point: The male hormone testosterone has been shown to play a significant role in the weakening of the perineal musculature. As a result, dogs being treated for these hernias are routinely neutered as well to prevent a recurrence of the problem.

The Nervous System

The nervous system, made up of specialized tissues and organs that originate electrochemical charges and transmit them to and from every organ system in the body, helps to regulate and coordinate the bodily functions required for life and to provide an environmental awareness. The main anatomical components of the system include the brain, which serves as the main control center for the entire system, the spinal cord, which acts as an information superhighway for nerves coursing to and from the brain, and nerve fibers, which interact directly with the tissues and organs. Groups or bundles of nerve fibers coursing together are referred to as nerves.

Nervous impulses are generated by sudden changes in electrolyte ratios of sodium and potassium along the membranes of neurons, the nerve cells that are the functional units of nerve tissue. The impulses then course down the nerve fiber to its end. Next, special chemicals released at the nerve tip transmit the impulse to an adjoining, predetermined nerve fiber, thereby keeping the impulse alive. In this way, a single impulse may be transmitted uninterrupted until it reaches its final destination.

The changes and disorders affecting the nervous system of older dogs reflect alterations in normal nervous anatomy, slowed or incoordinated impulse transmission due to age-related degeneration, or disruptions in electrolyte balance at the cell level, which can occur secondarily to kidney failure and a host of other disease conditions. In view of the important role of the nervous system, even a minor alteration or imbalance can have profound consequences for bodily function. Prompt response to the appearance of clinical signs relatable to nervous system disease, including seizures, behavioral changes, weakness or paralysis, incoordination, and reduced organ motility or contractility, is advisable.

Degenerative Disk Disease

Separating the spinal vertebrae of the back through which the spinal cord passes are special support structures called intervertebral disks, which serve as shock absorbers and points of flexibility along the spinal column. These circular disks are composed of tough, fibrous tissue surrounding a gelatinous center. With age, degeneration and subsequent hardening of this inner gelatinous mass may reduce the disk's ability to absorb shock. As a result, affected disks become quite susceptible to compression damage caused by routine activities such as running and jumping. Such damage can result in a rupture of the fibrous disk band and extrusion of the hardened center into the spinal cord space, placing pressure on the cord itself.

Dachshunds are especially susceptible to degenerative disk disease, as are cocker spaniels and poodles. Obese pets are also at higher risk for disk injury, owing to the increased pressure and work load placed upon the vertebral column. The two regions of that column most susceptible to disk degeneration and rupture are the neck and the lumbar area, located between the rib cage and the pelvis.

The severity of the clinical signs seen with degenerative disk disease is dependent upon the extent of the rupture. Partial or incomplete ruptures may put only mild pressure upon the spinal cord, leading to varying degrees of weakness and pain. Affected dogs are reluctant to move after the injury occurs and may cry or yelp when touched. When they finally decide to move, they may have difficulty walking due to weakness and incoordination resulting from the spinal cord pressure. Complete ruptures are accompanied by more serious clinical signs, depending upon the location along the spinal column at which the rupture occurred. Partial or complete paralysis of one or more limbs may result, and if damage to the spinal cord is extensive, all pain sensation in those limbs will be lost as well.

In most cases, diagnosis of degenerative disk disease can be made even prior to the occurrence of disk rupture and associated clinical signs through a physical examination and routine radiographs of the spine. If a rupture is suspected, radiographs will usually reveal the site(s) of disk collapse. To pinpoint the site and extent of a disk rupture, a special radiograph called a myelogram, in which an outlining dye is injected into the spinal canal, may be needed.

Treatment modalities for degenerative disk disease are chosen on the basis of the clinical signs exhibited. If mild weakness and incoordination are the only symptoms then conservative treatment consisting of strict cage rest and limitation of exercise for three to four weeks is usually prescribed. In more severe cases, in which the affected dog is having great difficulty walking yet still has feeling in the extremities, strict cage confinement in combination with anti-inflammatory drugs and other specific treatment is indicated. However, in dogs that experience sudden paralysis and loss of locomotion, together with a decrease or absence of feeling in the affected

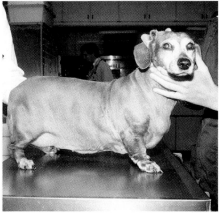

Obesity can be a major predisposing cause of disk rupture in older dogs.

limbs, immediate surgery is required to reduce the pressure placed on the spinal cord by the ruptured disk and prevent lasting damage to the cord. In general, the prognosis for recovery depends upon the extent of the rupture and the speed with which surgery is performed to relieve the pressure. Surgery performed within 24 hours of the onset of clinical signs yields the most favorable results.

If surgery proves unsuccessful, a quality-of-life assessment must be made to determine whether euthanasia should be considered. Special prosthetic devices are available that allow dogs paralyzed in the hind end by ruptured disks to ambulate by means of their front legs alone. Each case needs to be evaluated individually to determine the viability of such an option.

Several prevention methods can be employed to reduce the risk of back problems in an older dog. Certainly, placing an obese pet on a weight control program is of prime

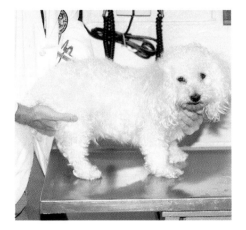

Dog with degenerative disk disease being supported at its hind end.

importance. Further, activities that could place undue pressure on the spinal cord, such as sudden bursts of running and jumping off furniture, should be discouraged. That applies especially to breeds predisposed to intervertebral disk disease, such as dachshunds. Last, surgery aimed at removing the gelatinous contents of disks that are apt to cause difficulties is a preventive measure that may be taken as well. It is especially effective in dogs that suffer from repeated bouts of clinical intervertebral disk disease.

Myelopathy

Myelopathies are degenerative diseases that strike the spinal cord and nerve fibers coursing throughout the body. They involve the gradual loss of myelin, the outer, conductive coating that surrounds certain nerve fibers. This loss impairs the fiber's ability to transmit nerve impulses. Common primarily in older, larger breeds of dogs, especially German shepherds, myelopathies are characterized by muscular incoordination, weakness, and atrophy. As the nerves innervating the hind legs are affected, a turning under or dragging of the hind feet may result. In fact, the hind limb weakness exhibited by some dogs with degenerative myelopathy is often mistaken for arthritis of the hips or spondylosis deformans of the spine. However, in this disease pain is rarely a factor.

Myelopathy is tentatively diagnosed on the basis of historical findings, clinical signs, and reflex testing. Dogs afflicted with this condition exhibit weak to absent reflex activity in their limbs. Electromyograms (EMG) may be performed as well to evaluate electrical activity associated with the muscle tissue of the body.

Unfortunately, because an exact cause of myelopathies—other than genetics—remains a mystery, there is no effective treatment to date. Vitamin therapy has been used in some instances to slow the progression of the disease, but motor incapacitation is inevitable.

Vestibular Disease

The vestibular system is a specialized portion of the nervous system found within the inner ear, brain, and spinal cord. Its duty is to maintain a state of equilibrium and balance. By communicating with the nerves supplying the eyes, limbs, and trunk, the body is able to coordinate the position and activity of those regions with movements of the head. Needless to say, any disruption in vestibular function makes it difficult for a dog to negotiate its environment. Classic clinical signs associated with vestibular disease include incoordination, circling, falling, rolling to one side or the other, head tilt, head tremors, abnormal eyeball movements, dementia, and nausea.

In older dogs the vestibular malfunction can result from ear infections, neoplasia, head trauma, and, rarely, hypothyroidism. Diagnosis of vestibular disease can often be made by clinical signs alone; however, a complete diagnostic workup is warranted to uncover the underlying problem. Once that is identified, treatment efforts can be aimed at the specific etiology.

Behavioral Changes and Canine Cognitive Dysfunction Syndrome (Senility)

Apart from the obvious physiological changes associated with aging, behavioral changes may occur with advanced maturity. Changes in behavior most often noted by owners of older pets include decreased activity, reduced environmental awareness and alertness, decreased appetite, decreased social interaction, and decreased willingness to obey commands. Most of these alterations can be traced to diminished sensory function, decreased nervous system efficiencies, pain, or the effects of underlying disease.

For instance, aggressive behavior in older dogs suffering from arthritis in the hips or even from periodontal disease can be sparked by slight contact with the painful region. In addition, the appearance of a house-soiling problem in older dogs is most likely due to age-related incontinence, musculoskeletal weakness, endocrine disturbances, or increases in dietary fiber, rather than to willed behavior changes. A thorough diagnostic workup is warranted whenever a change in behavior occurs, in order to detect or rule out underlying medical conditions that may be causing the problem.

Diagnosis of a behavioral problem begins with a thorough evaluation of the behavior's history, including time of onset, progression, and any distinct pattern of behavior that has developed. Certainly a complete physical examination and a laboratory workup are warranted as well, to rule out any medical conditions as causes. Once such conditions have been excluded, attention can then be focused on management of the specific behavioral problem.

In elderly dogs, separation anxiety can become a major instigator of behavioral challenges. This syndrome is characterized by constant barking or howling, inappropriate eliminations, or destructive behavior when a pet owner is away from home or separated from the pet in any way. It is an instinctive behavior of sorts. Dogs are pack animals by nature, and they strive for constant companionship. If their companion leaves for any reason, anxiety and frustration may occur. In addition, in older dogs these vices tend to be compounded by physiological changes and loss of sensory awareness associated with aging.

Separation anxiety attacks are often precipitated by some action performed by pet owners when leaving the house. By rattling car keys, turning off the television, or directing departing words to the pet, they can trigger an anxiety attack. Interestingly, such attacks and associated behavior usually occur within 15 minutes of the separation; then they subside. Owners may leave for a few short minutes, only to return and find their house and furniture disarranged and soiled. Fortunately, this feature of separation anxiety can prove to be useful in its management.

In the attempt to manage separation anxiety in an older dog, punishment is rarely effective, and it should be avoided. In fact, to a dog suffering from separation anxiety, the attention afforded by punishment seems better than no attention at all. Remembering the underlying cause of the anxiety attack, direct your efforts at modifying the dog's environment to break any associations that may set off an attack and to impart the secure feeling associated with companionship.

First, identify and discontinue all behavioral routines that may alert the dog to an impending departure. In fact, dogs are by nature creatures of habit, breaking routines is an effective way of managing many other behavioral problems in addition to separation anxiety. Next, implement a training schedule lasting four weeks. During this period, stage departures as often as possible, staying no more than 30 seconds each time, until the anxious pet becomes accustomed to you leaving and feels secure in knowing that you will return. As progress is made, the lengths of the absences can be slowly increased.

Leaving televisions and radios on may afford an otherwise anxious pet a feeling of security. Providing a replacement companion in the form of another pet or even a full-time pet-sitter is another option available for the treatment of this behavioral disorder. In cases of separation anxiety that prove especially difficult to manage, medications may be prescribed by a veterinarian to help calm an overanxious pet. These particular drugs, however, need to be used with caution in older dogs, which may be taking other medications or suffering from underlying medical conditions as well.

Fear of thunder or loud noises may become noticeable in older dogs, and it can become a significant source of stress and unacceptable behavior patterns. Frightened pets may become destructive or eliminate inappropriately. In addition, irrational behavior could lead to self-inflicted injury as the dog attempts to flee the source of discontent. Avoid direct efforts to hold and comfort a frightened pet, since they will only reinforce the behavior and could lead to human injury. Instead, attempt to distract the dog's attention through play, and muffle the frightening sound by turning on a television or radio. Drug therapy can help dogs that cannot be soothed by other means.

Antianxiety medications and drug therapies have other uses as well. Most pet owners are familiar with the saying "You can't teach an old dog new tricks." Since dogs are creatures of habit and routine, attempting to curb undesirable behavior by means of retraining or obedience techniques can be difficult in an elderly pet. When repeated attempts to change an undesirable behavior through training fail, low doses of specific antianxiety medications during the reprogramming process may provide the assistance needed. As one might expect, administration of these drugs for such a purpose requires the direct supervision of a licensed veterinarian.

Like humans, older dogs can experience senile changes resulting from degeneration of the central nervous system. Senility in dogs, also known as cognitive dysfunction syndrome, is characterized by disorientation, confusion, and failure to recognize familiar people and places. Other signs of this condition include frequent pacing, repetitive licking of a particular area of the body, increased vocalizations, excessive daytime sleepiness or nighttime wakefulness, and apathy toward life in general.

A number of conditions are believed to lead to the development of senility. They include hypothyroidism, epilepsy, tumors, and other structural diseases of the brain. Another popular theory espouses the notion that senility has its origin in oxygen deprivation to the brain caused by heart or lung disease. The involvement of these diseases and conditions has yet to be conclusively proved, however.

Senility in older dogs is diagnosed by ruling out all other potential causes of the abnormal behavior. No specific treatment exists for this disorder, but clinical trials are being performed with new drug agents that may significantly improve the clinical signs associated with senility. Until they become available, certain management measures may be taken to compensate for the decrease in neurologic awareness. These can include altering the dog's environment to allow for easier navigation, increasing the frequency of grooming sessions to make up for diminished self-grooming, and providing mental stimulation in the form of play, exercise, and obedience training on a daily basis.

The Endocrine System

The endocrine system consists of a vast network of glands and organs throughout the body that produce and secrete substances called hormones. Hormones, in turn, regulate body functions and reactions vital for life and coordinate complex interactions between the various body systems.

Hormones are made either of protein or of special fatty substances known as steroids. They are usually named according to their gland of origin (thyroid hormone) or their action (antidiuretic hormone). Both protein and steroid hormones are secreted directly from their parent gland into the bloodstream, where they are conveyed to the specific organ or tissue on which they exert influence. The amount of hormone required for a desired effect is precise; excesses or deficiencies can lead to manifestations of endocrine disease. Such disruptions become more likely as a dog matures, because of normal, age-related wear and tear on the endocrine glands, and because of the predisposition of older pets to neoplasia and immune-related dis-

Obesity caused by hypo-thyroidism in a cocker spaniel.

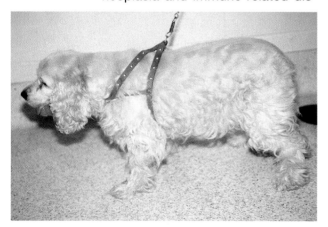

orders affecting those glands. In addition, because a single hormone may affect a number of different body systems and functions, an endocrine disease can produce a wide variety of clinical signs.

Hypothyroidism

Thyroid hormone is produced by the thyroid gland, located near the base of the neck. This hormone enhances the utilization of nutrients and oxygen within the body, thereby driving metabolism. If a deficiency of thyroid hormone occurs, a state of hypothyroidism is said to exist.

The causes of hypothyroidism in older dogs include immune system disorders, iodine deficiencies, and malfunctions of the pituitary gland. Certain breeds seem to have a predisposition to hypothyroidism. For example, the incidence of this disorder is greater in cocker spaniels, Dobermans, dachshunds, and golden retrievers than in other breeds. Interestingly, toy breeds rarely suffer from this condition. In addition, intact female dogs are less likely to suffer from hypothyroidism than are their neutered counterparts.

Clinical signs associated with this hormone deficiency include lethargy, exercise intolerance, and intolerance to environmental temperature fluctuations. Affected dogs tend to gain weight despite poor appetites. Over half of all older dogs suffering from hypothyroidism exhibit skin and hair coat changes.

A generalized thinning of the coat takes place, the skin thickens and tends to "droop," and secondary seborrhea usually rears its ugly head. Advanced cases of hypothyroidism can also lead to vision loss, nerve disorders, and joint inflammation if not treated properly.

Hypothyroidism can be easily diagnosed with simple blood analyses and thyroid stimulation tests. Treatment entails the daily administration of synthetic thyroid hormone in liquid or tablet form. To ensure that the dosage is correct, retesting should be performed within six weeks after treatment has begun. In most cases, supplementation will need to continue for the remainder of the dog's life.

Hyperadrenocorticism (Cushing's Disease)

Hyperadrenocorticism is a disease characterized by an overproduction of glucocorticosteroid hormones by the adrenal glands. These hormones regulate the utilization of carbohydrates, proteins, and fats within the body. In addition, they play an important role in maintaining water and electrolyte balance through their influence upon the kidneys. Finally, certain types of these hormones possess potent anti-inflammatory properties, exploited by veterinarians for the treatment of canine allergies and inflammatory conditions.

In Cushing's disease, the overproduction of glucocorticosteroids usually occurs secondary to a

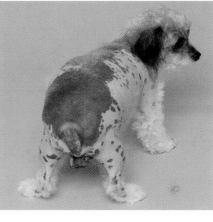

Hair loss associated with hypothyroidism.

tumor affecting either the adrenal glands or, more commonly, the pituitary gland, located at the base of the brain. A syndrome resembling Cushing's disease can be induced by indiscretionary, long-term administration of corticosteroid medications to dogs suffering from chronic allergies, arthritis, or immune system disorders.

Clinical signs of Cushing's disease include noticeable increases in food and water consumption, increased urination frequency, exercise intolerance, hair loss, dry seborrhea, skin pigmentation, and diminished muscle mass and tone throughout the body, resulting in a characteristic "pot-bellied" appearance. Ulcerations of the corneas of the eyes may appear as the disease progresses, and because high doses of certain types of corticosteroids can be immunosuppressive, secondary infections involving the skin and urinary bladder are not at all uncommon. If a tumor of the pituitary gland is involved, seizures and other neuro-

Skin lesions associated with Cushing's disease.

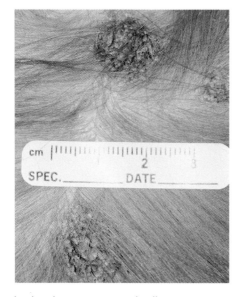

logic signs may gradually appear as the tumor slowly increases in size.

As mentioned previously, indiscriminate, long-term administration of certain types of corticosteroids to dogs with allergies, arthritis, and autoimmune diseases can eventually lead to the development of clinical signs similar to those of Cushing's disease. Further, since the artificial source of corticosteroids causes the dog's own body to halt the production of its own, natural corticosteroids, abrupt cessation of long-term steroid therapy can lead to an Addisonian crisis, a life-threatening condition. As a result, pets taking steroids for a medical condition should never be taken off them abruptly, but slowly weaned from them over weeks or months.

Definitive diagnosis of canine Cushing's disease can be made with blood tests specific for this disorder. In addition, radiographs may reveal adrenal gland lesions, helping to confirm a diagnosis. Treatment of hyperadrenocorticism is dependent upon the location of the tumor. Chemotherapy utilizing a special drug called mitotane is used to reduce the amount of steroids being produced by the adrenal glands. During the initial weeks of treatment, close monitoring for adverse reactions to the drug is required. In conjunction with this treatment, antibiotic therapy may be prescribed to combat secondary bacterial infections. In addition, diets that are high in protein should be fed to these dogs to help counteract the protein loss caused by excessive corticosteroid activity. Finally, surgical removal of the inciting tumor can be attempted in select cases. This procedure is usually reserved for cases that fail to respond to medical management.

Hypoadrenocorticism (Addison's Disease)

Hypoadrenocorticism is in effect the opposite of Cushing's disease, with inadequate amounts of corticosteroids being produced by the body. Special types of corticosteroids, called mineralocorticoids, are vital to the maintenance of fluid and electrolyte balance within the body. Deficiencies in these hormones, as with Addison's disease, can have serious consequences.

Tumors, infections, autoimmune diseases, toxins, and indiscriminate treatment with corticosteroids can all predispose older dogs to Addison's disease. Clinical signs include loss of appetite, weight loss, vomiting, diarrhea, and dehydration. Profound weakness occurs as disruptions in sodium and potassium balance within the body lead to heart and muscle fatigue. In severe instances the heart rate may slow to such an extent that circulatory collapse and shock result.

Definitive diagnosis of Addison's disease is achieved by evaluating the ratio of sodium to potassium in the blood. Obvious increases in potassium levels with commitment decreases in sodium levels, in the presence of clinical signs and electrocardiogram analysis, are diagnostic for Addison's disease.

If Addison's disease is suspected, treatment should start immediately, even before a final diagnosis has been achieved. Treatments with intravenous fluids and mineralocorticoids will normalize fluid and electrolyte levels in the body. Once stabilized, dogs afflicted with primary Addison's disease will require periodic injections with mineralocorticoids for life. For dogs whose Addisonian signs are due to an abrupt cessation of glucocorticoid therapy, reinstituting such therapy and then gradually reducing the dosage given over three to four months should help prevent a recurrence of the crisis.

Diabetes Mellitus

Insulin, the hormone secreted by the pancreas, is primarily responsible for regulating the utilization of glucose by the cells of the body. If production of this hormone is interfered with by disease or injury involving the pancreas, diabetes mellitus occurs. Older female dogs seem to be at greater risk of developing this disease than their male counterparts.

Clinical signs associated with diabetes mellitus result from the inability of the cells of the body to receive energy in the form of glucose. High levels of glucose in the bloodstream spill over into the urine lead to increased urinations and thirst. Excess glucose in the blood can also infiltrate the lens of the eyes and lead to cataracts and blindness. Diabetes mellitus can reduce the body's resistance to infection, and affected dogs often suffer from secondary bacterial infections of the skin and urinary tract. Damage to small blood vessels caused by the effects of the insulin deficiency can lead to kidney disease and gangrene of the skin and outermost extremities. Finally, in response to the lack of available glucose, protein and fat reserves are called upon by the cells of the body for conversion into energy. That often causes profound weight loss and muscle atrophy. As fats are broken down for energy, substances called ketones are produced and accumulated within the body. If the levels of ketones become too elevated, liver damage, pronounced nervous system depression, and pH imbalances can result. Dogs with such severe, complicated cases of diabetes mellitus may exhibit vomiting, diarrhea, breathing difficulties, dehydration, and depression to the point of unconsciousness. Cases exhibiting such symptoms are medical emergencies and should be treated accordingly.

Diagnosis of diabetes mellitus is based upon observing clinical signs, detecting consistently elevated glucose levels in the blood and urine, and ruling out other causes of similar clinical signs, such as Cushing's disease, kidney disease, and diabetes insipidus. Treatment of diabetic dogs suffering from severe clinical signs includes intravenous fluid therapy, pH modifiers, and insulin infusions. Close monitoring is required to ensure that blood glucose levels do not fall too low as a result of the insulin administration and lead to convulsions.

For dogs exhibiting uncomplicated signs of diabetes mellitus, insulin injections are indicated to help normalize glucose utilization within the body. Such injections which can be administered at home, must be performed in strict accordance with the veterinary treatment protocol. You need to keep accurate daily records reflecting morning urine glucose values as determined by special test strips, insulin amounts given, appetite characteristics, exercise activity, and any behavioral abnormalities. In addition, follow a strict feeding schedule and use special diets prescribed for diabetic dogs. Diabetic dogs that are overweight need to reduce as well in order to derive maximum insulin effectiveness.

When administering insulin injections to a diabetic pet, begin by gently swirling the insulin vial to mix the contents. Do not shake the vial; that could damage the insulin molecules within the solution. Next, swab the injection top of the vial with a cotton ball and alcohol and then, using the insulin needle and syringe, withdraw the desired amount of insulin from the vial. Once the proper dosage has been prepared, lift or "tent" the skin over either shoulder or hip region. Firmly insert the needle into the skin and underlying tissue, taking care not to penetrate the opposite side of the skin. Once the needle is inserted, withdraw the plunger slightly. If no blood is visible, administer the injection and withdraw the needle. Dispose of the needle and syringe properly.

Be aware that injecting too little insulin is better than too much. If too much insulin is given, a condition known as insulin shock could result. Clinical signs of this condition are related to low blood sugar and include trembling, weakness, incoordination, and, in advanced cases, seizures. If treatment instructions are closely followed, severe insulin shock should not be a problem. To be on the safe side, however, always keep a bottle of pancake syrup or honey handy for quick oral administration should signs of insulin shock appear. Two tablespoons of either fluid should be enough to replenish blood sugar levels and dissipate early signs of shock.

Diabetes Insipidus

Diabetes insipidus is an endocrine disease caused by a deficiency of a hormone that influences the kidneys and regulates the water content of urine. Insufficient amounts of that hormone, produced in the brain and called antidiuretic hormone (ADH), or lack of response to its effects by the kidneys can be caused by diseases that affect those organs. Clinical signs associated with diabetes insipidus include increased urination, excessive water consumption, and urinary incontinence.

Diagnosis of this disorder is achieved by ruling out other causes of urinary incontinence and increased urinations, and by using special tests that measure levels of antidiuretic hormone in the blood and gauge the kidney's ability to respond to ADH administration.

If it is deemed that too little ADH is being produced by the brain, treatment for diabetes insipidus will consist of daily administration of a natural or synthetic ADH supplement to correct the deficiency. On the other hand, if the fault lies in the kidney's ability to respond to the hormone, treatment tends to be more difficult. In general, special drugs called thiazide diuretics can be given to help counteract the effects of the

disease. Regardless of the treatment method used, providing affected canines with free access to fresh water at all times is vital to prevent disease-induced dehydration.

Hyperparathyroidism

The parathyroid glands, which are closely associated with the thyroid gland in dogs, produce a hormone that is responsible for increasing calcium levels in the blood by drawing stores of this mineral from bone and other regions of the body. Hyperparathyroidism is a condition initiated by a deficiency of calcium within the bloodstream. That can result from feeding diets that are high in phosphorus (nutritional hyperparathyroidism), such as all-meat diets, or, more commonly in older dogs, from increased phosphorus levels in the body caused by kidney disease. When such a calcium deficiency occurs, the parathyroid glands respond by secreting large amounts of hormone, which draws calcium out of bone in an attempt to normalize blood calcium levels. Over time, the bones become weakened and prone to stress injury (see Metabolic Bone Disease, p. 73).

Clinical signs of this metabolic disease in older dogs include lameness, weakness, bone deformities, and spontaneous fractures. A definitive diagnosis can be made by evaluating blood calcium levels and relating them to historical or other laboratory findings (history of poor diet or kidney disease; laboratory evidence of kidney disease). Treatment for nutritional hyperparathyroidism includes dietary modification and calcium supplementation. Unfortunately, there is no effective treatment for hyperparathyroidism caused by kidney disease except treatment of the kidney disease itself.

The Digestive System

The digestive system converts food into essential nutrients needed by the body for growth, maintenance, and repair. It also provides a means of eliminating waste material from the body. The organs of the digestive system begin with the teeth, tongue, and salivary glands. Chewed food is directed by the tongue to the esophagus, a long, muscular tube that moves food down into the stomach through a series of muscular contractions. In the stomach, the food is mixed with acids and enzymes as the process of digestion continues. From the stomach, the food moves into the small intestine, where special enzymes complete its conversion into smaller nutrients that can be absorbed into the body. Undigested waste is then shunted into the large intestine, or colon, where water is either added to or reabsorbed from the waste material. Finally, it is expelled through the rectum and anus to complete the digestive cycle.

In addition to the organs mentioned there exist, accessory digestive organs that produce or store enzymes, acids, and hormones essential to the digestive process: the pancreas, the liver, and the gall bladder.

Periodontal Disease

Periodontal disease is probably the most prevalent health disorder among older dogs today. Characterized by tender, swollen gums, halitosis (bad breath) and tooth loss, periodontal disease, if left untreated, has been proved to cause secondary heart and kidney disease in pets.

It originates with the accumulation of food particles and bacteria on the tooth surfaces. This accumulation, commonly known as plaque, eventually mineralizes and form a hard dental calculus on the surface of the tooth. Appearing as brown to yellow crusts, these calculi may extend up under the gumline, where they create gum inflammation and pain. Left untreated, the inflammation and infection associated with periodontal disease weaken tooth support structures and lead to tooth loss.

As a rule, smaller breeds of dogs such as Yorkshire terriers, poodles, and Chihuahuas are more prone to quick formation of dental calculi than are larger breeds, and they need more frequent preventative dental care. Diet also plays an important role in the development of plaque and subsequent periodontal disease. Older dogs fed dry dog foods are less susceptible to this disease than dogs fed moist or semimoist rations. Further, diets that contain excessive phosphorus, such as those consisting primarily of meat and meat by-products, have also been linked to this disorder. Metabolic diseases such as hypothyroidism can lead to gingivitis and subsequent periodontal disease. Tumors involving the gum or base of the tooth or the skull in the facial region can also play a role in the development of this disease. Finally, any disease that weakens the immune system and causes undue stress can predispose a dog to tooth and gum disease.

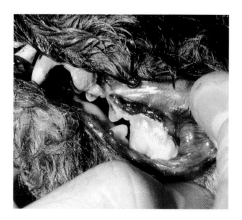

Severe periodontal disease.

The effects of periodontal disease, in addition to those above, include gagging or retching as inflammation peaks within the mouth. Gum recession, bleeding, and tooth recession arise as the disease reaches advanced stages. Infected teeth can form abscesses and may lead to secondary sinus infections, characterized by subsequent nasal discharges or draining tracks on the sides of the face. To make matters worse, bacteria from infected teeth and gums can gain entrance to the bloodstream and seed the body with infectious organisms. Two of the most common organs affected are the heart and the kidneys. In the heart, bacterial infections usually involve the heart valves, which subsequently deteriorate to the point of congestive heart failure. In the kidneys, infection and inflammation caused by bacteria can lead to fibrosis and eventual kidney failure.

Treatment of periodontal disease entails a thorough scaling and polishing of the teeth while the pet is under anesthesia (see Dental Care, p. 32). This procedure is essential to remove the calculus from under the gumline and to relieve any pockets of pus that may have formed near the base of the teeth. In addition, teeth that are excessively loose may form a nidus for infection, and they are generally removed to allow for drainage and medication. Dogs suffering from moderate to advanced cases of periodontal disease are also placed on antibiotics to combat bacteria that may have spread within the body.

Ulcers

Ulcers are caused when the loss or breakdown of the protective mucus covering the inner surfaces of the digestive tract allows stomach acids, bile acids produced in the liver, or toxins to erode and digest the lining of the stomach and intestines. In aged canines, the most prevalent causes of ulcer formation include metabolic and endocrine diseases such as kidney disease and Cushing's disease, respectively; neoplasia; stress associated with acute or chronic illness; and prolonged therapy with certain types of drugs, such as anti-inflammatory agents. Symptoms exhibited by dogs with digestive system ulcers include loss of appetite, lethargy, vomiting, and diarrhea. If the ulcerations are extensive, they may cause bleeding, which may manifest itself as black, tarry stools or blood-tinged vomitus or both.

Ulcers are diagnosed on the basis of clinical signs and physical exam findings, as well as radiography and endoscopy. Treatment efforts are geared to correcting any underlying cause, and drugs are administered to reduce stomach acid secretions or to replace the protective coatings over the ulcerated areas.

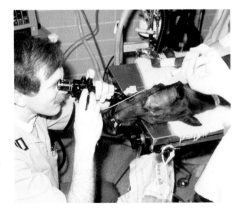

Endoscopy is an effective means of diagnosing gastrointestinal ulcers.

Gastric Dilatation-Volvulus Complex (GDV)

Gastric dilatation-volvulus complex, also known as GDV or bloat, is a life-threatening disease that affects the stomach of large, deep-chested breeds, such as German shepherds and Saint Bernards. Characterized by gross enlargement of the stomach due to gas accumulation, with subsequent twisting or rotation of the stomach around its axis, GDV can quickly lead to an impairment of circulation to all the vital organs within the abdomen, with deadly consequences.

One of the major causes of GDV is believed to be the rapid ingestion of large amounts of food and water, followed soon after by exercise. This combination leads to excessive gas formation, and the stomach begins to dilate and eventually rotates. That seals all the outlets that could allow the gas to escape. Even more gas is produced as the distressed stomach churns and secretes more digestive juices in response to the irritation. In rare instances GDV in older dogs is instigated by tumor development involving the stomach or adjacent organs. In those instances the anatomy of the stomach and its outlets is altered by the tumor growth, and it is difficult for gas and stomach contents to escape.

Clinical signs of GDV include a noticeably distended abdomen, vomiting and dry heaves, excessive salivation, and rapid breathing. Early on, affected dogs exhibit restlessness due to pain, and as the disease progresses and circulation is impeded, collapse and shock often occur.

A diagnosis of GDV can usually be made from the clinical signs. Confirmation can be achieved with radiographs, which are also useful in determining the extent of stomach rotation that has occurred. Treatment must be instituted immediately if the pet's life is to be saved. The gas is evacuated from the stomach through a stomach tube or by inserting a needle through the abdominal wall into the stomach. Intravenous fluids, antibiotics, and steroid compounds are administered to combat the shock that often accompanies GDV. The prognosis for recovery in dogs with GDV is very guarded, and it is dependent upon the length and extent of circulatory impairment.

Because this condition tends to recur with great frequency, surgery is often performed once the dog's condition has been stabilized. The ultimate goal of the surgery is to permanently affix a portion of the stomach wall to the inner abdominal wall in order to prevent rotation should the bloat recur, and to address any other factors, such as tumors that may be contributing to the disease development.

Preventive measures can thwart the development of GDV. Dividing the daily ration into smaller portions and increasing the number of daily feedings is one means of prevention. Further, discourage exercise

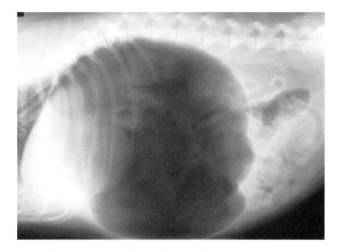

and rigorous activity for at least 90 minutes following a meal. At the first hint of trouble, contact a veterinarian. The sooner a bloat is treated, the greater is the chance of complete recovery.

Radiograph revealing a grossly enlarged stomach, associated with GDV.

Pancreatitis

The pancreas is an organ responsible for the production of essential digestive enzymes that break down foodstuffs into usable, absorbable units within the small intestine. It is also the site of production of the hormone insulin, which is vital for the conversion of glucose to energy.

Inflammation involving the pancreas is termed pancreatitis. In older dogs, pancreatitis can result from tumors, intestinal obstructions, infectious diseases, and, most commonly, dietary indiscretions (consuming garbage or food that is not normally a part of the diet). In the last case the pancreas overproduces digestive enzymes in

91

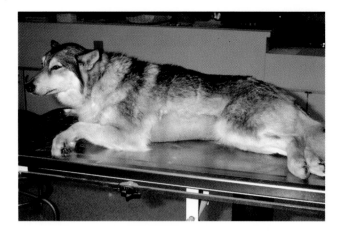

Postsurgical recovery for a patient suffering from bloat (GDV).

response to the indiscretion and begins to digest itself.

Signs of pancreatitis include loss of appetite, excessive salivation, vomiting, diarrhea, depression, and severe pain in the portion of the abdomen located on the right side, just behind the rib cage. The pain often leads dogs to assume a characteristic "praying" posture, with the elbows placed on the ground and the hind end elevated in an effort to relieve the pain. If the pain and inflammation caused by pancreatitis are severe, shock and death can result. In other instances, repeated bouts of pancreatitis can damage the insulin-producing cells of that organ and cause diabetes mellitus to develop.

Pancreatitis is definitively diagnosed by evaluating the blood for elevations in levels of amylase and lipase, two pancreatic enzymes. Radiography, ultrasonography, and endoscopy are also useful in determining the severity of the disease and in ruling out obstruction or neo-

plasia as the underlying cause of the flare-up.

Dogs experiencing only mild pancreatic inflammation caused by improper diet often recover when denied all food and water for at least 24 hours. This action effectively signals the pancreas to slow the release of its enzymes. In severe cases of pancreatitis, it is imperative that all food, water, and even oral medications be discontinued for at least 48 hours. Intravenous fluids will be required as well to prevent dehydration during this time. Additionally, antibiotics, pain relievers, and medications designed to reduce pancreatic secretions are usually employed to prevent secondary complications.

Upon recovery, dogs should be maintained on a dietary ration that is low in calories and easily digestible to reduce the work load placed on the pancreas (see Nutrition for Your Older Dog, p. 9). Avoid feeding table scraps and nonapproved treats, since even a small amount could precipitate a life-threatening attack. If your pet is overweight, increasing exercise levels and promoting weight loss will reduce its susceptibility to subsequent flare-ups.

Liver Disease

The primary function of the liver is to render harmless the toxic byproducts of the digestive process. In addition, this organ provides a storage site for vitamins and other nutrients and helps remove aged red blood cells from circulation and process them. It is also the production site for specific blood proteins and bile acids, the latter of which are stored in the gall bladder and secreted into the small intestine when needed to aid in digestion.

Inflammation involving the tissue of the liver is termed hepatitis. The causes of hepatitis in older dogs are varied, and they most often include diabetes mellitus, infections, heart disease, accidental poisonings, malnutrition, and neoplasia. Extensive or repeated damage to liver tissue can also lead to a condition known as cirrhosis, in which the liver shrinks in size as normal liver tissue is replaced by nonfunctional scar tissue.

Clinical signs associated with liver disease include loss of appetite, vomiting, diarrhea, fever, and jaundice, a yellow-orange discoloration of the skin, mucous membranes, and tissues caused by elevated levels of bile pigments in the bloodstream. In long-standing cases of hepatitis, ascites, or fluid accumulation within the abdomen, results from impaired circulation through the liver. Further, blood clotting disorders and anemia may arise owing to disruption of the liver's normal functions, and, as ammonia levels in the bloodstream rise as a consequence of the liver's inability to properly process this toxin, severe neurologic signs, including seizures, can result.

Diagnosis of liver disease is based upon clinical signs, elevated serum levels of liver enzymes, or the demonstration of an enlarged or shrunken liver on radiographs or ultrasound. Special liver function tests and liver biopsies may be required to determine the extent of the disease and yield, a prognosis.

Treatment for liver disease is aimed first at eliminating any underlying causes and second at promoting healing of the affected liver tissue. If these goals are achieved, the prognosis for recovery is good, since the liver does have the capacity to regenerate itself and replace cells lost to disease.

General treatments to control the symptoms and syndromes caused by liver disease include intravenous fluids and antivomiting medications, vitamins, and, in severe cases of anemia, blood transfusions. Once these and other acute problems caused by the liver impairment have been brought under control, affected dogs should be started on an easily digestible diet with high nutritional value. In addition, oral antibiotics may be prescribed to limit the number of ammonia-forming bacteria within the digestive

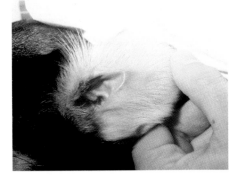

Dogs with severe liver disease usually show signs of jaundice.

system. Fluid buildup in the abdomen can be treated with special medications and by keeping sodium levels in the diet to a minimum. Finally, in chronic cases of liver disease, anabolic steroid therapy may be employed to stimulate appetite and overall metabolism.

Intestinal Parasitism

Fortunately, the incidence of intestinal parasitism is much lower in older dogs than in younger ones. However, it can still pose a threat to an elderly dog if poor preventive management is practiced by its owner.

Gastrointestinal parasites can rob an older dog of much-needed nutrition and weaken the immune system, predisposing it to other diseases and conditions. In addition, the parasites can cause vomiting, diarrhea, dehydration, and, in some instances, anemia if left unchecked. Fortunately, diagnosis of internal parasitism is usually easily achieved, and antiparasitic medications specific for the parasites involved can be administered to rid the body of an infestation. In older dogs, the most significant intestinal parasites likely to be encountered are roundworms, hookworms, whipworms, tapeworms, and protozoal parasites.

Roundworms, or ascarids, are thick-bodied, cream-colored worms that inhabit the small intestines of affected dogs. Living within the lumen of the intestine and absorbing nutrients through its body wall,

an adult roundworm sometimes reaches seven inches in length! In small numbers they rarely cause anything more than mild intestinal upset; however, if enough worms are present, bowel obstruction, with its associated consequences, can occur. Immature roundworms can also damage internal organs, since they may migrate to the lungs, liver, and other body organs, causing inflammation along the way.

Each adult female worm sheds thousands of eggs per day into the environment via her feces. Once the eggs are consumed by a dog, larvae hatch from them and may begin a migration through the bowel wall and into the liver and lungs. Once they reach the lungs, the maturing larvae are coughed up and swallowed again by the dog, so that maturation is completed within the small intestines. Unique signs associated with roundworm infestation include a distended abdomen, vomitus filled with worms, coughing, and even neurologic signs if migration was extensive.

The next type of parasite that may be found in the intestines of older dogs is the hookworm. Hookworms are much smaller than roundworms, yet they can cause severe enteritis. Instead of remaining within the lumen of the intestine, these worms attach themselves to the intestinal lining with their sharp mouthparts and suck blood and nutrients from it. A large worm burden within the intestines can lead to severe inflammation and irritation, in addition to significant blood loss.

Like roundworm eggs, hookworm eggs are passed out into the environment via feces. However, once they are outside, larvae hatch from them and search out a canine host. The larvae may be accidentally ingested by an unsuspecting dog. Alternatively, they may bore through exposed skin in order to gain entrance to the body. If that happens, intense itching and reaction can occur at the site of penetration. Once inside the body, the larvae migrate to the small intestines, where they reach maturity.

Unique symptoms associated with hookworm infestations include tarry or bloody stools and weakness, with pale mucous membranes as a result of anemia. In addition, footpads and other regions of the skin that were penetrated by hookworm larvae can appear reddened, bleeding, and infected.

Whipworms are slender parasites that inhabit the large intestine of infested dogs. Unlike roundworms and hookworms, these parasites do not undergo tissue migration, but are transmitted from dog to dog by fecal-oral contamination. Whipworms rarely cause severe disease in their canine host; in fact, they may reside within the large intestine of older dogs without causing any problems, except the outward signs of a dull, lackluster hair coat and mild weight loss. However, when a dog is suffering from intermittent bouts of diarrhea,

whipworms should always be on the list of potential causes.

Tapeworms are flat, segmented worms that can reside in the small intestines of dogs. They are undoubtedly the most common intestinal parasites in older dogs. The most prevalent species of tapeworm in dogs, *Dipylidium caninum,* uses the flea as an intermediate host. Tapeworm egg baskets that are shed in the feces of infected dogs are consumed by flea larvae, inside which they hatch into immature tapeworms and begin development. When a mature flea infested with a tapeworm is accidentally ingested by a dog during chewing or self-grooming activities, the tapeworm is released into the dog's small intestine, where it attaches itself to the intestinal lining and completes its maturation.

Dipylidium infestations are usually easily diagnosed by the presence of white to tan tapeworm segments in the feces and on the hair coat just beneath the tail. Infestations with this particular species of tapeworm rarely cause significant health problems. Affected dogs may have a dull hair coat and experience mild weight loss, but diarrhea is rarely a factor with *Dipylidium* in the older dog. Treatment for these worms involves the use of antiparasitic drugs designed specifically for tapeworms, and flea control.

Elderly pets can harbor other tapeworms besides *Dipylidium.* They are usually contracted when the dog consumes raw meat or is exposed to wild animals. Unfortunately, these tapeworms are not quite so innocuous as the flea tapeworm, and they can cause noticeable weight loss and enteritis. In addition, many of them pose a significant health threat to humans as well. If such a tapeworm infestation is diagnosed upon microscopic examination of the feces, prompt treatment should follow.

The next type of parasite that may cause clinical signs of enteritis in older dogs is the coccidium. Coccidia belong to a special group of microscopic parasites called protozoans. Transmitted from dog to dog by fecal-oral contamination, these parasites inhabit the small intestines and can cause diarrhea and dehydration. In general, however, this type of parasitism rarely causes problems in older dogs.

Finally, giardiasis is a disease that sometimes strikes older dogs. It is caused by the intestinal parasite *Giardia lamblia,* a protozoal parasite like the coccidia. These organisms are transmitted through special cysts that are shed in the feces of infected dogs. Once ingested by another dog via contaminated feces or drinking water, the cysts develop into mature organisms within the small intestine and can cause enteritis. Oftentimes, the diarrhea caused by *Giardia* is intermittent. It usually exhibits a characteristic yellow, foamy appearance.

Diagnosis of intestinal parasitism is achieved through microscopic examination of a representative stool sample. As a rule, the fresher the stool sample examined, the better the chances of accurate results. In the cases of tapeworms, whipworms, and protozoans, multiple samples may need to be tested.

Numerous effective medications are available for the treatment of the various intestinal parasites of dogs. It is important to be aware that different medications and treatment regimens are required for each parasite mentioned. Attempting to treat suspected parasitism without first identifying the exact organism involved can be futile. For that reason, and to ensure complete elimination, treatments for intestinal parasites in older dogs should be performed only by licensed veterinarians.

Preventing intestinal parasitism in the first place is preferable. Strict sanitation measures can help protect both dog and owner from exposure to potential parasites. Disposal of fecal material within 24 hours will keep potentially infective eggs from contaminating the dog's environment. In addition, prompt treatment of any confirmed parasitism will also keep environmental contamination from becoming excessive. Complete flea control and denial of access to raw meat or wild animals will help keep tapeworm infestations to a minimum. Finally, one of the most effective methods of intestinal parasite prevention is the administration of a once-a-month heartworm preventive medication that also exhibits activity against intestinal parasites.

Since heartworm prevention should be given to all older dogs in any case, that is a convenient way to solve two problems at the same time (see Internal Parasite Control, p. 21).

Hemorrhagic Gastroenteritis

Hemorrhagic gastroenteritis is a life-threatening condition that can be rapidly fatal if not treated promptly. Characterized by an explosive onset of bloody diarrhea, it can quickly cause dehydration, depression, shock, and toxemia. It is most often seen with dietary indiscretions or bouts of pancreatitis. Toxins produced by bacteria in an irritated gut cause such extensive inflammation that overt bleeding within the digestive system results. Toxins and bacteria may then permeate the hemorrhaging blood vessels and gain entrance into the body, with serious consequences.

Diagnosis of hemorrhagic gastroenteritis is based on history and clinical signs, as well as exclusion of other causes of digestive system disturbances. Treatment consists of intravenous fluids to control dehydration, high levels of antibiotics to combat infection, and high dosages of steroid anti-inflammatories and other medications to control shock and counteract the effects of toxemia.

Colitis

The term colitis refers to inflammation of the large intestine. Typified by tenesmus (straining to defecate) and loose stools often containing blood and mucus, colitis often becomes a recurring challenge in the older dog.

In seniors, the most common causes of colitis are dietary indiscretions and psychological stress that lead to bacterial overgrowth within the colon. Rectal polyps, tumors, foreign bodies, allergies, metabolic diseases, and immune system disorders can also cause colonic inflammation, as can intestinal parasites such as whipworms and coccidia.

Diagnosis of colitis is made on the basis of historical, physical, and stool findings. Special laboratory tests (including allergy testing), radiography, and endoscopy may all be employed to determine the underlying cause of the colitis. In cases that prove especially difficult to diagnose, a colonic biopsy may also be needed.

As with most other digestive system diseases, treatment depends on the underlying cause. The diarrhea associated with colitis can often be controlled with antibiotics to eliminate any bacterial overgrowth and with bismuth subsalicylate mixtures to provide a protective coating and reduce inflammation.

Dietary management is an important factor in the treatment of colitis. Upon initial flare-ups, bland, easily digestible diets can help calm most irritated colons. As in humans, chronic, recurring bouts of the disease can often be effectively managed by increasing the fiber content of the ration to promote normal, regular bowel movements. If a food allergy is diagnosed, a hypoallergenic diet is the correct choice for dogs with colitis.

Anal Sac Disease

The anal sacs are anatomical structures located beneath the skin on either side of the anal opening. Their function is to produce a special fluid, quite odorous in nature, that serves as an identification marker for other dogs. Although the contents of these sacs are normally expressed with every bowel movement, many owners find, to their dismay, that their pet can also express them at will when stressed or frightened!

The material within the sacs has a tendency to become thick and gritty if not emptied on a regular basis. Poor emptying may occur secondarily to allergies and other sources of skin inflammation, diarrhea, constipation, parasites (such as tapeworms), and dietary changes. As the material becomes thicker with time, impaction and, ultimately, infection of the anal sacs occur.

Signs associated with anal sac impaction and infection include constant licking at the inflamed sacs, scooting the hind end along the ground (in an attempt to express the sacs), and localized pain. In advanced infections, draining tracts of pus may issue from the skin surrounding the sacs.

Impactions of the anal sacs are treated by manual expression.

Infected anal sacs are first emptied in the same way, then instilled with antibiotic ointment. Oral antibiotics may also be used to expedite recovery. These procedures should be performed only by a qualified veterinarian. Sedation or anesthesia may be necessary if the discomfort is too great.

Contrary to what some believe, routine manual expression of healthy anal sacs is not advisable, since, if performed improperly, it can actually cause inflammation and promote impaction. Instead, most cases of anal sac disease can be prevented through proper diet. Increasing dietary fiber will promote more frequent bowel movements and thus more frequent emptying of the sacs. In addition, encouraging weight loss in obese dogs through dietary changes will also reduce the incidence of problems. Finally, for recurring bouts of anal sac infection, surgical removal of the sacs is a viable option.

The Integumentary System

The skin and hair coat of the dog protect its body from intrusion by foreign invaders or substances, provide sensory awareness of the surrounding environment, act as storage sites for water and nutrients required by the body, and help regulate body temperature. The sebaceous glands within the skin secrete oils (sebum) onto the skin, and these substances lubricate and moisturize the outer body surface and hair coat and inhibit the growth of bacteria or fungi on the skin surface. In addition, ancillary structures such as claws and pads aid in locomotion and defense and help reduce the stress on bones and joints.

The hair cycle and seasonal shedding ensure that the hair coat remains fresh and vibrant. Triggered by increases or decreases in daylight, peak shedding periods for dogs occur during the spring and fall months. For canines that spend the majority of their time indoors, shedding may become a year-round phenomenon.

As dogs grow older, alterations in normal skin anatomy and function occur with greater frequency and can predispose to disease. In addition, the skin and hair coat are affected by old-age diseases and disorders that originate in other organ systems. As a result, the appearance and integrity of the integument of older dogs can provide valuable insight into their overall health and well-being.

Allergies Affecting the Skin

Next to fleas, allergies account for most itchy skin and hair loss in older dogs. An allergy is caused by an exaggerated immune response to a foreign substance within or on the surface of the body. Allergies may develop at any time during a dog's life, with the severity of the reaction varying with the individual. Allergies that manifest as skin dis-

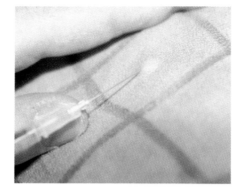

Intradermal skin testing for allergies.

ease in elderly dogs are classified into five main groups: inhalant allergies, flea allergies, contact allergies, drug eruptions, and food allergies.

Inhalant allergies, also called atopic dermatitis, are among the most prevalent of all allergies in older dogs. Most onsets occur in youth, with the condition persisting into maturity. Grass and tree pollens, molds, dander, house dust, and hair are some of the substances that can cause atopic dermatitis in dogs. Signs of this type of allergy include rubbing the face, licking and chewing at the feet, scratching behind the elbows and shoulders, and symmetrical hair loss. Small red bumps may be noticeable on the skin, and secondary skin infections due to the biting and scratching are not at all uncommon. Because the ear canals are extensions of the skin, ear infections are a recurring problem in dogs with inhalant allergies.

Diagnosis of atopic dermatitis is based upon a history of the clinical signs (seasonal versus nonseasonal), response to treatment, or

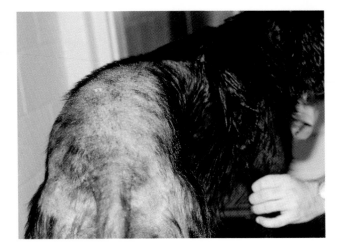

Profuse hair loss associated with a flea allergy.

be a satisfactory substitute for steroid therapy in many dogs. Antihistamines such as diphenhydramine have a calming effect on an itchy pet and help reduce the agitation caused by the allergy. Omega-3 fatty acids are a select group of fatty acids derived from cold-water fish oil that have been shown to exhibit anti-inflammatory effects in dogs. In some cases of atopic dermatitis, the response to these natural oils is so great that they suffice as the sole method of treatment! Excellent advances in medicated shampoos and sprays have also been made in recent years. New oatmeal-based shampoos and sprays used one to three times weekly provide excellent relief from itching and skin inflammation associated with atopic dermatitis. In addition, topical treatments containing effective antimicrobial agents such as chlorhexidine are now available for use on dogs with secondary bacterial skin infections occurring in conjunction with their allergies. Hyposensitization injections provide yet another approach to treating atopic dermatitis in older dogs. These injections contain extracts of the substance(s) identified by intradermal testing as the cause of the atopic dermatitis. A series of injections given at predetermined intervals can often condition the body to ignore the presence of the offending substance, and thereby the allergic response is reduced. Good success rates have been reported by some veterinari-

allergy testing. That testing may involve actual injections of potential allergy-causing agents into the skin and observation for reactions (intradermal testing) or, less reliably, evaluation of blood serum samples for antibodies to offending agents.

Inhalant allergies can be treated with topical shampoos and medications, steroid anti-inflammatory drugs, antihistamines plus fatty acids, hyposensitization injections, or a combination of two or more of the above. Traditionally, steroid anti-inflammatory drugs have proved most useful in the control of the clinical signs associated with inhalant allergies. However, because long-term continuous use can have deleterious side effects, especially in older dogs, one or more of the other modes of treatment should be considered. Oral administration of antihistamine medications, in combination with Omega-3 fatty acid therapy and regular medicated shampoos, can

ans using this method of therapy. However, results vary depending upon geographic location, the particular veterinarian performing the testing and treatments, and the individual pet involved.

Flea allergies, contact allergies, drug eruptions, and food allergies: Apart from the itching and irritation caused by the mechanical action of fleas biting the skin, the itching and hair loss seen with a flea allergy are the results of an allergic response by the body to flea saliva deposited into the skin. The clinical signs of a flea allergy tend to localize along the back, (especially near the base of the tail), hips, and rear legs. Diagnosis is determined by the presence of fleas on the dog and the distribution of clinical signs. Obviously, flea control is the treatment of choice for this disorder. In addition, the same types of treatments used to control atopic dermatitis can help reduce clinical signs associated with flea allergies.

Contact allergies are immune responses by the body to noxious substances that come in contact with the skin. Common offenders include detergents, shampoos, sprays, insecticides, flea collars, carpets, bedding, and plastic bowls used for feeding. Clinical signs consist of redness and itching and swelling of the affected skin, especially at points of contact such as the face, abdomen, and feet. Diagnosis of a contact allergy is made from the type and location of the clinical signs, and by separating the dog from the suspected offending agent and observing for clinical improvement. Treatment is achieved by permanently removing the offending agent from the dog or the environment. When sprays, chemicals, or other topical agents cause the contact allergy, thorough rinsing of the skin and hair coat with water should be followed by the administration of prescribed topical antibiotics or anti-inflammatory medications to fight existing clinical signs.

Drug eruptions, characterized by intense itching or hives on the skin, can occur when a dog is allergic to a certain type of drug . An association between the appearance of clinical signs and the drug's administration confirms a diagnosis of this type of allergy. As one might expect, discontinuation of the drug in question will result in abatement of clinical signs.

The final category of skin allergies is food allergies. Today, as food allergies are being increasingly blamed for a wide variety of dermatological disorders in dogs, large numbers of pet food companies are marketing "hypoallergenic" diets to the unsuspecting public. In fact, the incidence of food allergies is not so great as those companies would like you to believe. Food allergies become suspect when other types of allergies have been ruled out as the cause of dermatologic disease in a pet. Symptoms associated with an allergy to food include itching, hair loss, hives, and facial swelling.

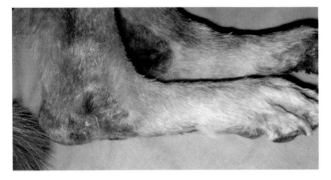

Allergic skin disease.

Diarrhea, vomiting, and other digestive system maladies may appear as well, and they can clue an alert veterinarian to a tentative diagnosis. An authoritative diagnosis is achieved through the use of food allergy trials, in which the dog is fed a diet of hypoallergenic ingredients. If a positive response is seen within six weeks, a food allergy is said to exist. The dog will be maintained on the special diet indefinitely, to prevent recurrence.

Seborrhea

Skin that is excessively flaky or oily is said to be seborrheic. Seborrhea occurs as a primary disease entity in certain breeds of dogs, such as cocker spaniels, Doberman pinschers, Labrador retrievers, and West Highland white terriers. More commonly this disorder occurs secondary to other diseases such as allergies, nutritional deficiencies, skin parasites, skin infections, and hypothyroidism.

Diagnosis of seborrhea in older dogs is based primarily upon clinical signs. Identification of the underlying cause is a essential to

Seborrhea.

effective treatment. In especially challenging cases, skin biopsies may be required to determine whether primary seborrhea is the definitive cause. Treatment of seborrheic skin includes medicated shampoos, nutritional supplements (including vitamin A derivatives called retinoids) and steroid anti-inflammatory medications. If the seborrhea is dry and flaky, moisturizing skin conditioners and fatty acid supplements may also be employed to eliminate the clinical signs. Finally, daily brushing will do wonders to overcome the effects of seborrhea.

Skin Calluses

Calluses affecting the elbows and ankle regions are quite prevalent in

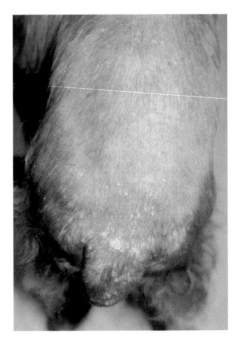

larger breeds of dogs as they age. Caused by friction from lying on and rising up from hard surfaces, calluses are unsightly, yet pose no real health threat. In some instances the callus may become so dry and cracked that a bacterial infection develops. Treatment with a topical antibiotic cream or ointment will readily resolve that problem. In addition, daily application of skin moisturizers, lanolin, or vitamin E cream to the callused areas may help soften the callus and promote hair regrowth. Finally, providing carpets, blankets, towels, or any other type of soft bedding for a pet to lie on is an effective way to support treatment efforts and to prevent the continued development of the calluses.

Hormonal Skin Disease

Many hormonal imbalances within the dog's body can manifest themselves as skin disease. For instance, hypothyroidism, diabetes mellitus, and Cushing's disease can adversely affect the skin and hair coat. Clinical signs of skin disease related to hormonal imbalance can include symmetrical hair loss, abnormal pigmentation, open sores and/or large scabs or crusts, and excessive thickening or thinning of the skin. Interestingly, itching is rarely a sign of hormonal skin disease unless the skin changes are accompanied by seborrhea or infection. Diagnosis of a hormonal disorder can be achieved through the use of appropriate laboratory tests. Of course, proper treatment

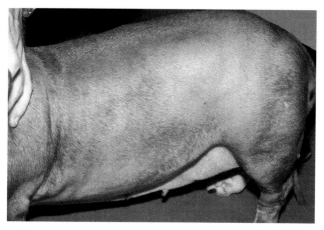

Hair thinning resulting from hormonal imbalances.

of the imbalance will lead to the resolution of clinical signs.

Another type of hormonal disease that affects primarily older dachshunds and cocker spaniels is acanthosis nigricans. Characterized by symmetrical hair loss, increased pigmentation, and thickening of the skin in the armpit and chest regions, this condition must be differentiated from skin allergies and thyroid hormone imbalances, which may cause similar symptoms. That differentiation can be achieved through skin biopsy. Treatment of acanthosis nigricans involves the use of steroid anti-inflammatory medications to reduce pain and inflammation, and antibiotics to combat any secondary infection. Aloe vera or vitamin E creams can be applied topically to soothe and comfort irritated skin.

Autoimmune Skin Disease

Although relatively rare, skin diseases caused by malfunctioning immune systems are serious when they do occur in older dogs. With autoimmune diseases such as pemphigus and lupus, cells and tissue comprising the skin and mucus membranes are attacked and damaged by the immune system, leading to characteristic blistering and ulcerating lesions. Following diagnosis through the use of skin biopsies, management of skin lesions caused by autoimmune disease is achieved using large doses of steroid anti-inflammatory medications. For more information on autoimmune diseases, see Autoimmune Disease, p. 105.

The Immune System

The immune system is a combination of specialized organs, cells, and chemicals that interact to protect the body from foreign invaders and neoplastic cells. Without it, the body would be quickly overcome and destroyed by a hostile environment. Although genetics plays the primary role in determining the strength and efficiency of this system, other factors such as good nutrition, reduced stress, and routine priming certainly contribute to the efficacy of the immune response.

Organs of the immune system include the bone marrow, the thymus, the spleen, and lymph tissue found throughout the body. The bone marrow is the origination site of the various immune system cells. The thymus gland, located at the base of the neck in young animals, plays an important role in the maturation of immune cells. It slowly regresses as a dog grows older. The spleen, located within the abdomen, acts as a filter and storehouse for blood and immune cells. Finally, lymphatic tissue and glands found throughout the body help filter foreign matter from lymphatic fluid and blood.

Cells of the immune system include neutrophils, monocytes, macrophages, and lymphocytes. Neutrophils are white blood cells that engulf and destroy bacteria that gain entrance to the body. Assisting the neutrophils are monocytes and macrophages, immune cells that consume not only bacteria, but viruses, fungal organisms, and foreign matter as well. Granulomas, which are firm masses commonly mistaken for tumors, consist of conglomerations of macrophages and other cells that surround and imprison foreign matter, preventing its spread within the body. Lymphocytes are the immune cells responsible for producing antibodies against disease organisms and foreign tissues. These cells require periodic priming through immunization to ensure that they are ready at all times to produce protective levels of antibodies, should an actual invasion occur. Certain types of lymphocytes are also responsible for destroying cancerous cells as they arise within the body.

Last, the immune system produces chemicals that aid in the

stimulation and modulation of the immune response and in the destruction of foreign invaders and tumor cells. Among these chemicals are interferon, interleukins, and complement. Much research is being devoted to the study of such chemicals and their immunologic effects, in hope of harnessing their awesome power for concentrated use in the treatment against cancer and other devastating illnesses.

Allergic Reactions

Allergic reactions result from overblown responses by the immune system to foreign organisms or substances that have gained entrance to the body or have attached themselves to it. These reactions can follow the administration of medications or vaccinations, exposure to environmental irritants, insect bite and stings, or the ingestion of certain foodstuffs or poisons. The extent of the allergic reaction depends on the amount of previous exposure to the allergy-causing agent and on the degree of the current exposure.

Clinical signs seen with mild to moderate allergic reactions include intense itching, hives, soreness, vomiting, swelling, fever, and lethargy. The signs may appear minutes to hours following exposure. Life-threatening allergic reactions, known as anaphylactic reactions, can arise within seconds of exposure, however, and can cause breathing difficulties, collapse, shock, and even death. An allergy to bee or wasp venom is one example of an allergic response that can turn anaphylactic if there was prior exposure.

Allergic reactions are diagnosed by the clinical signs and the timeliness of their onset. Treatment for mild to moderate allergic reactions includes antihistamines to halt the further progression of the clinical signs and steroid anti-inflammatory medications to reverse existing symptoms. In instances of anaphylactic shock, intravenous fluid therapy, large doses of antihistamines and steroids, and oxygen therapy are needed to counteract the deleterious effects of the reaction.

Autoimmune Disease

Like allergies, autoimmune diseases are caused by exaggerated responses of the body's immune system. However, instead of being directed toward a foreign substance or invader, an autoimmune response is mounted against the body's own tissues and organ systems. Owing to the immense power of the immune system, autoimmune diseases can devastate the health of a dog.

Pemphigus complex is a series of autoimmune diseases that can cause severe ulcerations, crusts, and blisters on the skin of dogs, especially around the mouth, lips, nose, and footpads. In addition, these lesions are often itchy and extremely painful. Because of the loss of skin integrity, secondary bacterial skin infections can complicate matters.

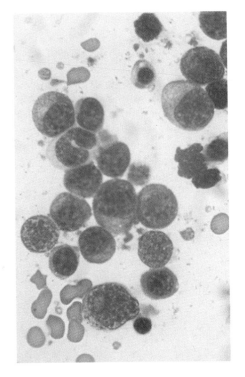

Lupus erythmatosis (LE) is another autoimmune disease that can cause skin lesions similar to those seen with pemphigus complex. In addition, it can damage other tissues and organs, including the blood, kidneys, muscles, and lymph nodes. Dogs with LE may also experience painful lameness as the immune system attacks the various joints of the body.

Autoimmune hemolytic anemia (AHA) is a condition in which perfectly healthy red blood cells are destroyed by the body in such numbers as to cause anemia (see Anemia, p. 56). Dogs suffering from AHA often experience extreme weakness and jaundice. Immune-mediated thrombocytopenia (IMT) involves a similar reaction by the body, but this time it is directed against the blood platelets. As a result, dogs with IMT experience blood clotting disorders, which can be life-threatening (see Bleeding Disorders, p. 57).

Finally, in rare instances the body's immune reaction to an invading organism or foreign substance may lead to organ damage, especially of the kidneys (see Pyometra, p. 68). Such damage can occur secondary to the formation of immune complexes, which consist of antibodies bound to the foreign invader, within the organ tissue. Organ failure may occur if the condition is not recognized and treated in time (see Metritis and Cystic Endometrial Hyperplasia Complex, p. 68).

Diagnosis of autoimmune disease is made through the evaluation of skin and organ biopsies, as well as specialized blood tests. Regardless of the type of autoimmune disease that is diagnosed, treatment utilizes extremely high doses of steroid hormones, which have a suppressive effect on the immune system. In especially difficult cases, other drugs that modulate and suppress the immune system, such as azathioprine and gold salts, may be used in conjunction with the steroid hormones to create a remission. Removal of the spleen, the site of most blood cell destruction, can also help dogs suffering from AHA or IMT.

Immunosuppression

Interference with normal immune function can have serious health consequences. A suppressed immune system leaves the body susceptible to, among other things, invasion by infectious organisms and proliferation of neoplastic cells. A certain degree of immunosuppression can occur as a result of the aging process, hence the increased susceptibility of older dogs to infectious diseases and cancer. In addition to aging, other sources of immunosuppression are certain viral diseases (parvovirus), stress, chronic disease (kidney failure), and bone marrow disorders. Endocrine disturbances such as hypothyroidism and Cushing's disease can also significantly reduce the effectiveness of the immune response. Finally, radiation and certain types of drugs, including steroid hormones and chemotherapeutic agents used to treat cancer, can leave the body susceptible to a variety of diseases because of their immunosuppressive effects.

A state of immunosuppression can be detected through laboratory analysis of the blood and bone marrow. If possible, treatment of the underlying cause of the suppression should be instituted as soon as a diagnosis is made. Depending upon the cause of the immunosuppression, anabolic steroids and other drugs designed to boost the body's immune system may be prescribed as adjuncts to therapy.

The Eyes, Ears, and Nose

Sensory function enables a dog to react to, and interact with, its environment. The senses operate in coordination with other organ systems to optimize their efficiency and to protect them from harm. Unfortunately, as aging takes its toll, the diminution of overall sensory function may decrease the efficiency of organs and impair the elderly dog's ability to cope with its environment.

The Eyes

The canine eye is designed to perceive generalized forms and images rather than distinct features. In fact, the visual acuity of the dog is similar to that of a human at sunset. Contrary to popular belief, all dogs have the ability to see in color, though their sense of color is not so vivid or well developed as humans'. As with the other senses, aging takes its toll on vision as well. Reduced sensitivity of the nervous endings in the eyes, in combination with anatomical changes in other ocular structures, can result in diminished sight.

The anatomy of the eye is unique. A large portion of the outer surface of the eyeball is covered and surrounded by a special membrane, pink in appearance, called the conjunctiva. A nictitating membrane, or third eyelid, is also present at the inside corner of each eye. Designed to protect the eye

The retina,
optic disk,
and tapetum
as seen
through an
ophthalmo-
scope.

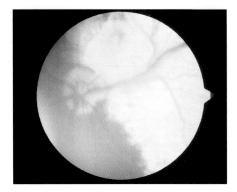

during aggressive encounters, this lid often protrudes over the surface of the globe in times of dehydration and cachexia as well. The clear, transparent membrane covering the front portion of the eye is called the cornea. As light passes through the cornea, it is directed through the pupil formed by the colored iris, which regulates the amount of light allowed into the eye. The lens of the eye, stationed just behind the iris, gathers light and focuses it on the retina lining the back wall of the eye. It is here that light is converted into nervous impulses. Those impulses, sent to the brain along large nerves, result in a visualized, perceived image. The tapetum is a layer of pigment that also lines the rear surface of the inner eye. This reflective layer improves dogs' night vision and is responsible for the characteristic green glow seen when light is shined into their eyes.

Glaucoma is a serious disease characterized by an increase in fluid pressure within the eye. In older dogs, glaucoma can develop secondary to lens luxations, cataracts, inflammation, and allergies. In some dogs, glaucoma is an inherited trait that may not appear until later in life. Glaucomatous eyes appear reddened and inflamed, with blue, hazy corneas and dilated pupils. Blindness may also result from pressure damage to the retina. In severe cases, the affected eyeball becomes noticeably enlarged and painful.

Diagnosis of glaucoma is confirmed by direct pressure readings taken with special instrumentation. Owing to the destructive nature of this disease, treatment aimed at reducing the pressure within the eye should be instituted without delay. Drugs designed to draw fluid out of the eye and back into the bloodstream will be used initially for that purpose. In addition, other medications that control the amount of fluid present within the eye will be used for long-term management. Anti-inflammatory drugs can also be employed to reduce the pain and inflammation associated with this disorder. When a luxated lens is causing the increase in pressure, or when the glaucoma cannot be effectively controlled with standard medications, surgery may be the only way to provide relief and preserve sight.

Cataracts and Lenticular Sclerosis: Cataracts are opacities of the lens that, in older dogs, can develop secondary to eye trauma, infections, or diabetes mellitus. The amount of visual impairment caused by the opacity is directly proportional to its maturity. In addition to mechanically obstructing vision, cataracts can also predispose the affected eyes to lens luxations and glaucoma.

True cataracts must be differentiated from another common condition in maturing dogs, lenticular sclerosis. Caused by a hardening of the lens material, it differs from true cataracts in that light can still penetrate the discolored lens, so that visual function is preserved. The two conditions can be differentiated by a trained veterinarian using a special instrument called an ophthalmoscope.

Treatment of cataracts involves surgical removal of the affected lens. That is accomplished by entering the eye and removing the lens intact. Alternatively, ultrasound is used to shatter the lens into smaller pieces, which are then extracted from the eye with specialized instruments inserted into the globe. Once the offending lens is removed, vision usually returns. If desired, lens implants or replacements can also be utilized in dogs to sharpen visual acuity even further.

Keratoconjunctivitis sicca (KCS; dry eye) is an eye disease that affects the cornea and conjunctiva. Caused by a reduction in tear production, KCS can dry the corneal surface and cause tissue damage and ulcerations. If it is left unmanaged, blindness can occur as a result of the corneal changes. Symptoms of KCS include a green, mucoid discharge in and around one or both eyes. Ulcers forming on

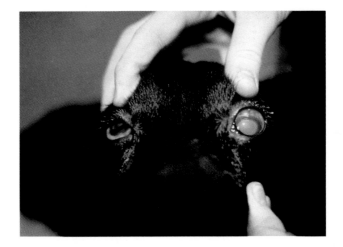

the surface of the corneas because of dryness cause redness and pain in the affected globes. If the KCS has been present for an appreciable time, dark pigments may have begun to infiltrate the cornea. It is they that can eventually lead to loss of vision.

Although KCS can be an inherited disease, especially in certain breeds such as cocker spaniels, schnauzers, and Yorkshire terriers, most cases that arise in later years are acquired. Causes of KCS in older dogs include hypothyroidism, diabetes mellitus, autoimmune disease, and chronic eye infections. Additionally, indiscriminate use of certain medications, such as sulfa drugs, can inhibit tear production and predispose to KCS.

Special tests designed to measure tear output are used to diagnose KCS. Treatment consists of tear replacement drops, applied to the eyes several times a day, and antibiotic/anti-inflammatory drops

Severe ocular changes associated with glaucoma.

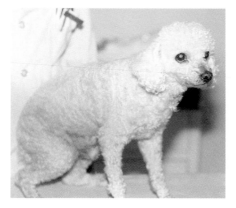

Cloudy eyes caused by lenticular sclerosis.

or ointment to combat infection and inflammation. As adjuncts to those treatments, drugs designed to stimulate tear production may be utilized. A few drops of 2% pilocarpine added to a pet's ration can help stimulate new tear production. One of the newer, more exciting advances in the treatment of KCS is the discovery and use of the drug cyclosporine. Research has shown that this drug, used topically on the eyes, is often very effective in reversing the effects of KCS.

When the pigment changes to the cornea are extensive or when conventional medical treatment fails to halt the progression of the disease, surgical intervention may become necessary to preserve or restore sight.

Retinal degeneration and disease associated with aging can cause blindness in older dogs. For instance, progressive retinal atrophy (PRA), a hereditary condition, can strike middle-aged to older dogs and produce blindness over a period of several months to years.

Breeds that are predisposed to this condition include Gordon setters, Irish setters, poodles, Norwegian elkhounds, Labrador retrievers, collies, cocker spaniels, and malamutes. Characterized by a slow degeneration of the receptor cells composing the retina, PRA in its early stages often leads to night blindness. Affected dogs tend to fear or shy away from poorly lighted areas. As PRA progresses, it eventually creates complete blindness by causing the pupils to remain dilated and fail to respond to light.

Retinal function may also be partially or completely lost through underlying disease or injury, leading to blindness. For instance, glaucoma can place so much pressure on the blood vessels supplying the retina of the eye that secondary retinal degeneration results. Sudden acquired retinal degeneration (SARD) is another nonhereditary condition that can cause blindness in older dogs, yet its exact cause remains a mystery. Interestingly, this disease is often accompanied by an increase in thirst and in appetite. Infectious diseases such as ehrlichiosis, Rocky Mountain spotted fever, and fungal disease can also adversely affect the region of the retina where the optic nerve exits and lead to inflammation and subsequent loss of vision. In addition, neoplasms such as lymphosarcoma can infiltrate the retinas of older dogs and inhibit retinal function. Finally, trauma, immune-mediated diseases, and certain tox-

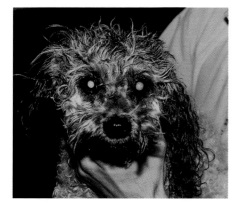

ins can injure the retina and induce blindness.

Diagnosis of retinal disease and degeneration is based on history, physical exam findings, and information obtained from ophthalmic examination of the retinas. In addition, an electroretinogram, which measures the electrical activity within the retinas, will provide a definitive diagnosis of retinal degeneration and retinal blindness. If a disease condition such as glaucoma, infection, neoplasia, or toxicity is suspected, other diagnostic testing procedures specific to those conditions may be required as well.

Unfortunately, there are no known treatments for PRA and SAR, and the prognosis for the restoration of sight in affected dogs remains grave. Other diseases involving the retina may respond favorably to treatments specific to the particular disorder; however, the longer such treatments are delayed or neglected, the greater are the chances of permanent loss of vision.

The Nose

The nose of the dog performs two basic functions. First, it filters and warms inspired air before it enters the respiratory tree. Special folds, called turbinates, within the nasal cavity can trap foreign debris and are rich in blood vessels that warm the inspired air. The second, and most obvious, function of the canine nose is olfaction, or smell. Air passing through the nose stimulates special hair-like receptors located at the top of the nasal cavities. Nerve fibers connected to those receptors carry the signal generated to that portion of the brain responsible for perceiving and recognizing odors.

Dogs' sense of smell, incredibly acute and precise, enables them to detect even the faintest scents in their surroundings. In fact, it is virtually impossible to mask an odor from a dog, hence this animal's effectiveness at scenting wild game, explosives, and controlled substances. Aside from its importance in the identification of people, animals, locations, and inanimate objects in the dog's environment, the sense of smell exerts a strong influence on appetite as well. Older dogs suffering from acute rhinitis or upper respiratory infections may refuse to eat if their sense of smell is impaired.

Rhinitis is an inflammatory condition involving the nose and nasal passages. The symptoms usually seen with rhinitis include nasal discharges, sneezing, and gagging

Cataracts can cause blindness in older dogs.

due to postnasal drip. Bacterial infections, fungal infections, nasal tumors, nasal foreign bodies, and trauma to the nasal passages are the most common causes of rhinitis in older dogs. Oftentimes infections leading to rhinitis occur secondary to disease-related immunodeficiencies or to immunosuppression caused by drug therapy (steroid therapy, chemotherapy). In long-standing cases of rhinitis, secondary fungal infections can arise. They are characterized by thick, mucoid discharges that may turn bloody if blood vessels within the nose become involved.

The underlying cause of rhinitis is diagnosed through the use of clinical signs, physical examination, radiographs, visual examination of the nasal passageways under sedation, or microscopic examination of the nasal discharge. Specific treatment will be determined by the underlying etiology. In cases of infection, properly selected antimicrobial therapy will help bring the rhinitis under control. In addition, anti-inflammatory medications may be employed to help eliminate the clinical signs. All disease conditions that may be stressing and suppressing the immune system must be properly identified and addressed if the cure is to be lasting. In select cases, surgery may be required to remove foreign bodies, such as grass awns or tumors, that are causing the inflammation.

Loss of smell: With advancing age, the nerve endings within the nose that are responsible for smell may slowly lose their sensitivity. That can also occur because of mechanical trauma to the nose or upon exposure of the sensory endings to chronic infections, toxins, and irritants found in the air.

As olfactory sensitivity diminishes, reduced appetites and behavioral changes often follow. Diagnosis of an olfactory disorder is accomplished through the use of special smell tests and through endoscopic examination of the nasal passages.

Unfortunately, there is no specific treatment that will restore olfactory sensitivity once it is lost. In an attempt to boost appetite, feed your pet rations with strong aromas to compensate for the sensory deficit. In addition, heating food prior to serving will increase its aroma. Dogs with olfactory deficits should not be allowed to roam outdoors, since their ability to sense danger via their nose is compromised.

The Ears

The upper range of canine hearing is thought to exceed 50,000 cycles per second, approximately twice the range of human hearing. High pitches undetectable to the human ear can elicit a response from a dog, often to the bafflement of its owner. Like the sense of smell, however, the hearing capacity of dogs diminishes with age as the nerve endings responsible for this function begin to wear out. In addition, various diseases and disorders can exacerbate hearing loss in older dogs.

The canine ear consists of three sections. The first is the external ear canal, which communicates directly with the outside environment. The middle ear, which is separated from the external ear canal by the tympanic membrane, or eardrum, acts as the bridge between this portion and the inner ear, which contains the nerve endings responsible for the sense of hearing. Disorders affecting any one of these regions can be responsible for partial or complete deafness in older dogs.

Ear Infections: The external ear canal is separated from the middle ear by the tympanic membrane, or eardrum. In dogs, this external portion of the ear can become infected with bacteria, fungi (yeast), or parasites. Clinical signs associated with an external ear infection include head shaking, itching, pain, and often an odorous discharge from the affected ears. Discharges from the external canal may become so profuse that hearing is adversely affected. Yellow to green discharges usually signify bacterial involvement, whereas brownish discharges are usually seen with yeast infections. Mixed infections are not uncommon. In the case of ear mites, a characteristic dry, black, flaky discharge indicates their presence.

Diagnosis of the causative agent can be made through microscopic examination of the discharge. The type of treatment prescribed will depend upon the extent of the infection and upon the organism involved. Antibiotics and antifungal medications, instilled directly into the external ear canal, will help clear up most infections. Ear mite infestations may be managed with antiparasitic medications. Since ear infections can occur secondary to other disease conditions such as hypothyroidism and skin allergies, identification and treatment of all underlying causes are essential to therapeutic success.

Like the external ear canal, the middle ear can become infected and inflamed, and hearing loss may result. Infections involving the middle ear usually result from long-standing infections of the external ear canal that penetrate the eardrum. The classic clinical sign associated with middle ear infection is a noticeable head tilt to the side of the affected ear. In addition, because nerves supplying the muscles of the face pass through the middle ear, paralysis of those muscles and subsequent drooping of the eyelids, cheeks, and lips may occur secondarily.

Diagnosis of a middle ear infection is confirmed by radiographing the suspected ear. Treatment consists of high doses of antimicrobial drugs to combat the infection and anti-inflammatory medications to alleviate the clinical signs. In severe cases, surgical drainage and medicated flushing of the middle ear canal may be needed to initiate healing.

Finally, because of direct communication with the middle ear, inner ear functions can also be disrupted by infections of the former. Additional signs of inner ear infections include loss of equilibrium, nausea, circling behavior, and abnormal twitching of the eyeballs, called nystagmus. Moreover, since the nerve endings responsible for hearing are located in the inner ear, dogs with untreated inner ear infections are at risk of developing nerve deafness. Diagnosis and treatment of inner ear infections are essentially the same as for the middle ear.

Nerve deafness: Infections are not the only source of deafness in older dogs. Nerve deafness can also arise secondarily to trauma to the ear, toxins, or treatments with certain types of medications. For instance, certain types of antibiotics called aminoglycosides may be prescribed to combat certain types of bacterial infections in older dogs. However, this class of drug can damage auditory nerves when used in high doses for extended periods of time. The damage is usually irreversible. As a result, veterinarians are especially cautious when selecting dosages and treatment durations of these drugs and others that may have similar effects upon hearing.

Diagnosis of nerve deafness is based upon history and special hearing tests. One such test, the brain stem auditory evoked response test (BAER), measures the brain's response to auditory stimuli and is quite helpful in the detection of hearing defects. The BAER can determine the extent of any such defect and pinpoint its location.

Unfortunately, no treatment exists for nerve deafness. Hearing aids designed especially for dogs are now commercially available, and they may improve hearing in select instances.

Cancer in Older Dogs

The term neoplasia refers to the uncontrolled, progressive proliferation of cells within the body. Bypassing the body's normal mechanisms for controlling growth, neoplastic cells reproduce at abnormal rates, often coalescing into firm, distinct masses called tumors. Neoplasia can be classified as either benign or malignant, depending upon the behavior of the cells involved.

Benign tumors consist of well-differentiated cells that divide and reproduce only slightly more rapidly than normal ones. Such tumors are slow-growing, well-demarcated, and noninvasive, rarely spreading to other parts of the body. They seldom pose a threat to life unless their sheer size interferes with the function of an adjacent organ or, as in the case of glandular tumors, their presence alters the production of vital hormones.

Conversely, malignant (cancerous) tumors experience frenzied growth, with uncontrolled spread (metastasis) to other organ systems. In addition, these malignancies tend to spread by means of finger-like projections far into the surrounding tissues (hence the name "cancer"), so that complete surgical excision is next to impossible. Growth and duplication of the malignant cells continue until the cancer kills the dog or until every malignant cell is removed or destroyed. Death from cancer occurs when vital organs and tissues are replaced or starved to death by the malignant cells.

Tumors are further classified according to their microscopic appearance and the body site in which they originate. To identify benign tumors, the suffix -*oma* is used. For example, a benign tumor affecting bone is referred to as an osteoma, and one affecting glandular (adenoid) tissue is called an adenoma. Malignancies, on the other hand, are given the suffixes -*carcinoma* (for malignancies involving epithelial or glandular tissue) and -*sarcoma* (for malignancies originating in other tissues of the body). For example, if the benign tumors referred to above were malignant, the correct terms would be osteosarcoma and adenocarcinoma, respectively.

Both carcinomas and sarcomas metastasize through the blood, with special affinity for the liver and lungs. Carcinomas also can spread via the lymphatic system, seeding lymph nodes with cancer cells along the way.

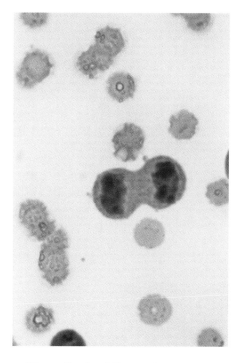

A dividing tumor cell.

The effect of the aging process on the development of neoplasia is not fully understood. One current theory is that as cells continue to replicate throughout life, the chances of genetic mutations or accidents resulting from one of the replications increase according to the law of averages. In addition aging may impair the body's ability to combat cancer-causing viruses or to counteract the effects of carcinogens, substances or agents known to induce genetic mutation in otherwise healthy cells. Examples of carcinogens are ultraviolet radiation from the sun, airborne hydrocarbons, certain drugs and medications, and thousands of other chemicals that may be applied to the skin or ingested by dogs. Finally, certain types of canine cancer, such as mammary carcinoma, can affect tissues and organs experiencing years of exposure to certain hormones produced within the body.

Nonspecific clinical signs of neoplastic disorders are listed in Table 10. Neoplasia must be differentiated from abscesses, granulomas, and fungal diseases, all of which can be mistaken for tumors. Extreme care must be taken when determining whether a true neoplasia exists, since inflammation and secondary infection often accompany tumors and can confuse the interpretation of test results.

Several methods and techniques are available to assist in the diagnosis of cancer in older dogs. Diagnostic protocol begins with a thorough history, an evaluation of clinical signs, and a physical examination. Tumors affecting the skin, oral cavity, and other mucous membranes can usually be readily detected upon careful physical inspection. In addition, tumors within the abdominal cavity can often be detected by skilled palpation of the abdomen. Endoscopy, radiology, ultrasonography, and cytology are generally the next diagnostic steps taken by the veterinary practitioner (see Diagnosing Illness in Older Dogs and Interpreting Laboratory Data, p. 36). One advantage of endoscopy is that if a tumor is indeed encountered, a biopsy of the neoplastic tissue can be immediately obtained through the instrument. A biopsy is by far the most reliable method of diagnosing neoplasia in dogs. In fact, biopsies obtained from tumors and surrounding lymph nodes are the only reliable means of determining whether a tumor is benign or malignant and whether metastasis has taken place. Laboratory evaluation of the cells in the blood, serum biochemistries, urine, and, in some instances, the bone marrow, may also assist in the detection of neoplasia that might not be apparent with other testing methods.

The type(s) of therapy chosen to treat a particular neoplasia is based upon six factors:

1. The type and characteristics of the neoplasm involved
2. The stage of its development, including the presence or absence of metastasis

---

Table 10
General Signs
Associated with Neoplasia

- Unexplained, pronounced weight loss
- Loss of appetite
- Chronic lethargy
- Firm, expanding lumps or masses
- Eating difficulties
- Breathing difficulties
- Persistent discharges
- Lameness
- Changes in urinary or bowel habits

3. The extent of spread and secondary organ involvement, if metastasis has occurred
4. The dog's overall physical condition, including any preexisting medical disorders
5. Prognosis for remission or cure
6. Financial and quality-of-life considerations

Treatment options for neoplasms include surgery, radiation therapy, chemotherapy, cryotherapy, and immunotherapy. Other forms of therapy, such as hyperthermia and antiplatelet therapy, do exist, but their use in veterinary medicine is limited. A combination of surgery, radiation, and chemotherapy is currently the most favored protocol for treating especially difficult malignancies in dogs. As one may expect, the earlier a cancer is detected, the greater are the chances for complete cure.

Surgery is by far the most common method of treating neoplasia. As a rule, "If it is removable, remove it." In most instances, if a primary tumor that has not metastasized can be surgically excised along with a margin of healthy tissue surrounding the mass (as a safety precaution), a complete cure can be achieved with the surgery alone. Confirmation of complete excision can usually be verified through biopsy. Surgery is also useful for partial excision of tumors that for some reason cannot be fully removed. When the size of the tumor is decreased, temporary relief from clinical signs associated with the tumor can be achieved, and

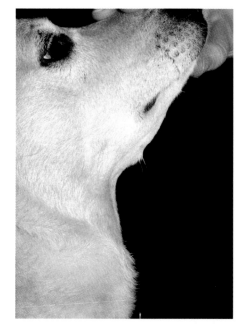

Enlarged lymph nodes in the neck of a dog.

the effectiveness of alternate treatments such as radiation therapy and chemotherapy can be improved. Finally, in extreme cases, surgical amputation of a limb may be required to eliminate a cancer. For example, osteosarcoma (malignant tumor affecting the bone) is such an aggressive form of cancer that, in almost all cases, amputation of the affected limb is the treatment of choice.

Radiation therapy utilizes ionizing radiation to kill malignant neoplasms. Radiation is administered to canine patients over a two- to three-week period either through the use of an externally produced radiation beam or by radioactive implant. It exerts its effect by destroying the genetic material within the cancer cells and thus eliminating their ability to multiply. Tumors that are especially sensitive to this type of treatment include early squamous cell carcinomas, mast cell tumors, and hemangiopericytomas. As a rule, radiation therapy is limited to tumors with definable margins and tumors that are slow to metastasize. As an adjunct to surgery, radiation therapy can be used to eliminate any microscopic neoplastic residues that have been unknowingly left behind by the surgeon.

A third mode of treatment, chemotherapy, involves the use of specific drugs designed to destroy neoplastic cells. Chemotherapy works on the premise that cancer cells are more sensitive to these chemical agents than are normal cells. This type of therapy is generally employed against tumors that have metastasized (or are suspected of doing so), cannot be totally removed by surgery, or are refractory to other forms of treatment. A few of the many chemotherapeutic drugs commonly utilized in veterinary medicine are cyclophosphamide, vincristine, cytosine arabinoside, and prednisone. The efficacy of chemotherapy is generally increased by the use of combinations of these drugs rather than just one. Each drug tends to have a unique effect on the cancer cell; therefore the neoplasia is attacked from multiple "directions" instead of only one. Further, combining drugs also increases the safety of the therapy, since it allows for the dosage of each drug to be lowered while treatment effectiveness is retained.

Possible side effects of chemotherapy in dogs include severe bone marrow depression, nausea, vomiting, and bleeding tendencies. Hair loss is less common in dogs than in humans. Fortunately, the side effects depend on the doses of chemotherapy administered; they can usually be controlled with proper adjustments of the dosage.

Treatment by means of freezing a tumor, or cryotherapy, is especially useful with masses involving the eyelids, mouth, and other areas where conventional surgery would be difficult. With cryotherapy, tumors are rapidly frozen to –20 degrees Celsius, then slowly thawed. This cycle is repeated two to three times, depending upon the type of tumor involved. Following such treatment, death and regression of the mass usually result.

Finally, a newer form of cancer therapy, immunotherapy, stimulates

Pigmented masses on the surface of the skin. Note the site where a biopsy was obtained.

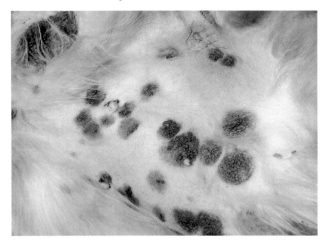

and supports the body's immune system in its fight against the disease. In theory, if immune-stimulating medications are injected into the body, the resulting immune response will destroy neoplastic cells. In actual practice, much research and refinement are still needed. However, one form of passive immunotherapy that shows great promise in the treatment of cancer utilizes monoclonal antibody technology. Monoclonal antibodies are immune proteins that have been artificially cultivated in the laboratory. Highly concentrated preparations of monoclonal antibodies are being used to attack specific cancer cells directly and to carry chemotherapeutic drugs directly to the cancer cells in order to increase their effectiveness. Once refined, this technology should revolutionize the way in which certain cancers are treated, both in dogs and in human beings.

When prognostic or financial considerations discourage treatment or call for its discontinuation, supportive measures may be instituted to improve the quality of the remaining days or weeks of the dog's life. Surgical removal of cumbersome masses, antibiotic therapy to control secondary bacterial infections, and anti-inflammatory drugs to alleviate pain and discomfort are palliative treatments that can be used in the terminal cancer patient. Of course, dogs experiencing a rapid decline in quality of life or intense pain due to cancer growth should be considered

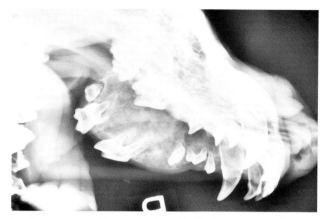

for humane euthanasia to eliminate their suffering.

Bone tumor affecting the upper jaw of a dog.

Select Types of Neoplasia in Older Dogs

Because of the number of different types of organs and tissues in the body, there are a multitude of types of neoplasms that can arise in elderly dogs. Certain types, however, appear more regularly than others. Tables 11 and 12 list some of the more common types and frequencies of tumors affecting older canines.

Adenomas affecting the skin account for the largest percentage of tumors in older dogs. There is no sex predilection for this type of tumor, and most occur in animals over nine years of age, particularly in cocker spaniels, dachshunds, miniature schnauzers, poodles, shih tzus, lhasa apsos, malamutes, Siberian huskies, and Irish setters.

Arising from glandular structures located within the skin (sebaceous glands), adenomas are cauliflower, wart-like growths that are pink to

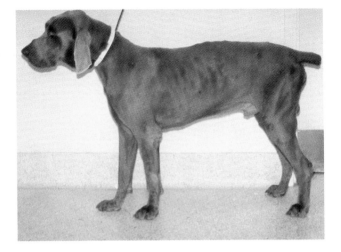

Multiple tumor nodules on the skin of an older dog.

sue, female dogs are more likely to develop such tumors than males. In fact, older female dogs that were spayed before their first heat cycle experience a dramatically reduced incidence of mammary cancer in comparison with females that were allowed to go through one or more heat cycles. However, when mammary tumors do arise in those females, and when they appear in male dogs, they are usually highly malignant. Breeds that seem especially susceptible to mammary neoplasia include Airedale terriers, Brittany spaniels, Irish setters, Labrador retrievers, poodles, springer spaniels, German short-haired pointers, and keeshonds.

These neoplasms can arise from a number of cell types within the mammary tissue itself, and they can be benign or malignant. Malignant mammary neoplasms grow quite rapidly; they tend to invade and cause inflammation in and around surrounding tissue. Metastasis to other organs such as the lungs, liver, bone, and kidney can occur as well. Mammary tumors appear as hardened, sometimes painful swellings usually involving the last two glands of the mammary chain, although the others may also be affected. Local lymph node enlargement, especially in the groin region, may become noticeable as well. A fluid discharge from the affected nipples may occur, and, if metastasis takes place, breathing difficulties, coughing, swollen limbs, vomiting, or diarrhea may arise.

orange in color, although some may be pigmented. The sites most commonly affected are the limbs, trunk, eyelids, and head. In most cases, adenomas are benign and pose little threat to the health of the pet.

Diagnosis of sebaceous gland adenomas is based upon physical appearance and biopsy test results. Treatment consists of surgical excision, cryotherapy, or heat therapy (actually burning off the tumor). Once removed, they rarely recur in the same location. However, they may appear elsewhere on the body. When multiple adenomas exist on a particular pet, treatment is sometimes forgone, unless the tumors appear to be growing extraordinarily fast or become ulcerated or traumatized.

Mammary adenocarcinomas, a type of mammary tumor, are the second-most frequent tumors affecting older dogs. Owing to hormonal influences on mammary tis-

The treatment of choice for any type of mammary tumor is surgical excision. That may involve simply removing the mass if only one location along the mammary chain is affected. In the case of multiple locations, the entire gland or a large portion thereof may need to be removed. Regional lymph nodes are removed as well if metastasis is suspected. Upon biopsy of the affected tissue, subsequent chemotherapy is recommended if the tumor is deemed malignant.

Lipomas, relatively common tumors in older dogs, can arise from fatty tissue anywhere in the body. Dachshunds, cocker spaniels, poodles, and terriers seem to be especially predisposed to this type of tumor. The most prevalent site of occurrence is the subdermal (beneath the skin) fatty tissue on the belly and chest regions. Lipomas present as soft, fluctuant round masses that are adhered tightly to surrounding tissue. As a rule, they rarely pose a health risk to a dog unless they become secondarily infected or reach such a size as to mechanically interfere with normal bodily functions. That can occur within the body cavities, where lipomas arising from fat adhered to body organs or from membranes lining the cavities form large masses that can impinge on surrounding organs.

Surgical removal is the treatment of choice for lipomas, yet they can be difficult to excise completely because they infiltrate into surrounding muscles and tissues. As a result, recurrences following surgery are not uncommon. In many instances, if tumor growth is minimal and there is little or no interference with normal bodily function, lipomas are left untreated.

The malignant form of fatty tumor, the liposarcoma, is rare in dogs, yet must be ruled out whenever a fatty mass is discovered. Veterinarians can distinguish lipomas from liposarcomas through cytology and biopsy procedures. If a malignancy is diagnosed, liberal surgical excision of the mass and a portion of the surrounding tissue is indicated in an effort to completely remove the cancer.

Malignant lymphoma/lymphosarcoma is another prevalent form of neoplasia in older dogs. It involves the neoplastic proliferation of lymphocytes in sites including the lymph nodes, digestive tract, skin, spleen, liver, and kidneys. Breeds prone to this type of tumor include boxers, Saint Bernards, cocker spaniels, German shepherds, beagles, and golden retrievers.

The primary clinical sign associated with malignant lymphoma typically is a generalized swelling of the lymph nodes throughout the body, especially noticeable in the neck, shoulder, hindlimb, and inguinal regions. Other nonspecific signs may appear as organ systems within the body become adversely affected.

Diagnosis of malignant lymphoma can be achieved through

Table 11
Common Tumors Affecting Older Dogs

Tumor Type	Tissue/Organ Affected	Primary Mode(s) of Treatment*	Comments
Adenocarcinoma	Perineum; anal sacs; thyroid; prostate; stomach and intestines; kidneys; ovaries	S,C, R, Cr	Malignant tumor associated with glandular organs
Adrenocortical adenoma	Adrenal glands	S,C	Accounts for 15 percent of all cases of Cushing's disease
Chondrosarcoma	Bone; nasal cavity	S, R, C	Malignant tumor of cartilage
Fibrosarcoma	Connective tissue beneath the skin; oral cavity; nerves	S, R, Cr	Tends to recur following surgery
Hemangiosarcoma	Spleen; blood vessels; heart	S, C, Cr	Increased incidence in German shepherds and other larger breeds
Hemangiopericytoma	Skin; blood vessels	S, R	Sensitive to radiation in early stages
Lipoma	Fatty tissue	S	Usually infiltrates into adjacent tissue
Lymphoma/ lymphosarcoma	Blood; lymph nodes; Intestines; spleen; liver; kidneys	C, I	Most common tumor affecting blood components in dogs
Mammary tumor	Mammary glands	S, C	One of the most common tumors affecting older, intact females
Mast cell sarcoma	Skin	S, R, C, Cr	Can be characterized by intense itching and allergic reaction
Melanoma	Skin; oral cavity	S, R	Often highly malignant and metastasizing
Metastatic bone tumor	Bone	S, C, R	Most often arises from mammary and prostate tumors
Metastatic liver tumor	Liver	S, C, R	Most often arises from stomach and intestinal adenocarcinomas; hemangiosarcomas
Metastatic lung tumor	Lungs	S, C, R	Most often arises from sarcomas; some carcinomas (mammary)
Osteosarcoma	Bone	S, C	Amputation is often treatment of choice

Table 11 Continued

Tumor Type	Tissue/Organ Affected	Primary Mode(s) of Treatment*	Comments
Papilloma; sebaceous adenoma	Skin; oral cavity; eyelids	S, Cr	Appears as wart-like growth on the skin and mucous membranes
Pituitary adenoma	Brain	S, C	Leading cause of Cushing's disease
Sertoli cell carcinoma	Testicles	S	Neutering is treatment of choice
Squamous cell carcinoma	Skin; bladder; oral cavity; nasal cavity	S, Cr	Lack of skin pigment and skin trauma can be predisposing factors
Transitional cell carcinoma	Bladder	S, C, R	Malignant cells may be detected in urine

*S - Surgery, C - Chemotherapy, R - Radiation, Cr - Cryotherapy, I - Immunotherapy

lymph node cytology and biopsy, radiographs of the abdomen and chest, and ultrasonography. Treatment involves chemotherapy and, in select cases, immunotherapy.

Melanomas are neoplasms that can affect the integument of older dogs, with a special predilection for the lips, tongue, gums, oral cavity, eyelids, and digits of the feet. Arising from pigment-producing epithelial cells, melanomas may be either benign or malignant. The degree of malignancy exhibited by these tumors seems to be directly correlated with their location. For example, melanomas involving the mouth and oral cavity tend to be more malignant than those affecting the digits or eyelids.

Male dogs seem to have a higher occurrence of this type of skin tumor than females. Breeds apt to develop melanomas, both benign and malignant, include cocker spaniels, chow chows, Doberman pinschers, Irish setters, springer spaniels, Boston terriers, Scottish terriers, and Chihuahuas.

Benign melanomas appear as darkly pigmented nodules or skin blotches with well-defined borders. Rarely do they exceed one inch in diameter. Malignant melanomas, on the other hand, appear as rapidly growing, often ulcerated masses or nodules that may or may not be pigmented and can reach greater sizes. These cancers often metastasize via the blood and lymph to various sites, including the liver, lungs, spleen, brain, spinal cord, heart, and bone.

As with other tumors, definitive diagnosis of a melanoma and its character is accomplished through biopsy and microscopic examination of the tumor. Radiography, ultrasonography, and lymph node

Table 12
Ten Most Common
Tumors in Older Dogs

Adenoma (skin)
Adenocarcinoma (mammary
   glands)
Lipoma (soft tissue)
Lymphoma (lymph nodes)
Malignant melanoma (oral
   cavity)
Osteosarcoma (bones, joints)
Hemangiosarcoma (skin,
   spleen)
Perianal adenoma (perianal
   glands, anal sacs)
Sertoli cell tumor (testicles)
Squamous cell carcinoma (skin)

biopsies may all be used to help determine the extent of metastasis if a malignancy is diagnosed. Treatment involves the surgical removal of the tumor and radiation therapy. Chemotherapy has proved of limited use in the treatment of malignant melanoma. Unfortunately, malignant melanomas usually have undergone metastasis by the time they are detected, and they tend to recur after surgical removal. The overall prognosis for cure is poor.

Osteosarcoma (OSA) is the name given to a highly malignant tumor involving the bones and joints of dogs. It is quite destructive in nature and metastasizes readily to other organs of the body, especially the lungs. Locally, bone destruction with infiltration of surrounding tissues occurs in most cases. Large breeds such as boxers, collies, German shepherds, Great Danes, Irish setters, and Saint Bernards seem to be most susceptible, with the incidence higher in males than in females. The most common site of involvement is the forearm, yet the tumor can also appear on the hindlimbs and even on the facial bones.

Clinical signs associated with OSA include limb swelling and lameness. Coughing, breathing difficulties, and other signs related to internal organ involvement may also be seen if metastasis has occurred. Diagnosis can usually be made from clinical signs and radiographs of the affected bones. Of course, biopsy evaluation is needed to confirm such a diagnosis.

Treatment for osteosarcomas involving the bones of the limbs involves aggressive surgical intervention, including amputation of the affected limb or special surgical techniques designed to preserve limb integrity while allowing for tumor removal. Chemotherapy should follow surgery to slow or eliminate metastatic disease. If chemotherapy is not instituted, over 90 percent of dogs diagnosed with OSA and treated with surgery alone will die within one year.

Hemangiomas and hemangiosarcomas are neoplasms that arise from the cells that make up the blood vessels. Common sites of occurrence include the spleen, heart, liver, and skin, although any organ in the body can be affected if metastasis via the blood takes place. Hemangiosarcomas tend to be very malignant and often ulcerate owing to rapid growth.

German shepherds, boxers, Scottish terriers, and Airedale terriers seem to have the highest incidence of this tumor type. Clinical signs associated with hemangiomas/hemangiosarcomas involving the skin include the appearance of soft, friable masses, usually on the chest or extremities. If the spleen or other internal organs are involved, the symptoms include weakness and depression, abdominal swelling, breathing difficulties, progressive emaciation, enlarged lymph nodes, and nosebleeds. Overt collapse and shock can occur because of excessive bleeding, typically from the spleen.

Diagnosis of these blood vessel tumors is based upon clinical signs and tumor biopsy results. Surgical excision or cryotherapy can be utilized on hemangiomas, with favorable results. Hemangiosarcomas, on the other hand, are a greater treatment challenge owing to their invasive and metastatic nature. Oftentimes, amputation of an entire limb may be required because of the tumor's invasiveness. Removal of the spleen is indicated in cases of splenic hemangiosarcoma. Chemotherapy can be employed postsurgically, though the prognosis for lasting recovery remains poor.

Perianal gland adenomas: Adenomas can also arise from modified skin glands in the region of the anus (perianal glands) and anal sacs of older dogs. Seen most often in dogs over 11 years of age, perianal gland adenomas are nine times more likely to occur in male dogs than in females, because the activities of these glands are normally modulated by sex hormones, mainly the male hormone testosterone. Interestingly, female dogs afflicted with Cushing's disease may be predisposed to these tumors because of the disease-induced elevated levels of testosterone that are being produced by the adrenal glands. Breeds that may be predisposed to this type of tumor include cocker spaniels, English bulldogs, Samoyeds, Afghans, dachshunds, German shepherds, beagles, Siberian huskies, shih tzus, and lhasa apsos.

Most tumors involving the perianal glands are benign; however, malignancy (adenocarcinoma) can occur, especially if the tumor involves the anal sac. As a result, diagnosis of these tumors should always include biopsy evaluation to determine their status. The treatment of choice for benign adenomas is castration, to remove the source of hormonal influence. In addition, in extensive cases, surgical excision, cryotherapy, and even radiation therapy can be used to expedite a cure. Therapy with estrogen compounds is often used to treat malignant adenomas, in addition to benign or malignant tumors in female dogs. Prognosis for recovery is good to excellent with benign tumors, guarded to poor with malignancies.

Sertoli cell tumors and other tumors involving the testicles are obviously limited to male dogs that have not been neutered. The incidence of this type of neoplasia is high in older dogs with retained testicles, that is, testicles that never descended into the scrotal sac and remain within the soft tissue of the groin region or in the abdominal cavity. That occurs because retained testicles are exposed to higher temperatures than testicles that have descended properly. That favors the formation of this particular type of tumor. Sertoli cell tumors are typically slow-growing, yet they can metastasize via the lymphatics to the lymph nodes and sometimes to other organs of the body, such as the kidneys, pancreas, and lungs.

Clinical signs associated with Sertoli cell tumors and other testicular tumors include enlarged testicles or inguinal/abdominal swelling, as well as other signs related to metastasis. Diagnosis is based upon clinical signs, history of retained testicles or inguinal herniation, and biopsy results. Treatment for testicular tumors involves surgical castration and removal of surrounding tissue. If the regional lymph nodes are thought to be involved, they should be removed as well. Chemotherapy, in combination with radiation therapy, may be employed following surgical recovery to combat recurrence and metastasis.

Squamous cell carcinomas (SCC) arise from the epithelial cells that constitute the skin. Areas of skin lacking pigment or subject to repeated trauma or irritation are especially susceptible to SCC development. The oral cavity, tonsils, lips, nose, and limbs are common sites of occurrence. In addition, SCC can involve the nails and toes, especially in dogs with dark hair coats. Breeds predisposed to SCC development include Labrador retrievers, giant schnauzers, boxers, Norwegian elkhounds, Pekingese, poodles, and Scottish terriers.

A squamous cell carcinoma may appear as a slightly raised mass, often with an ulcerated surface, or it may resemble a papule or wart. As a rule, these tumors slowly spread to other organs, yet usually readily invade surrounding tissue. Diagnosis is achieved through biopsy evaluation of the actual tumor. Surgery and cryotherapy are the most effective ways to treat SAC in older dogs.

In addition to the ten most common tumor types discussed above, other neoplasms that arise frequently in older dogs are fibrosarcomas, mast cell tumors, hemangiopericytomas, and bladder tumors.

Fibrosarcomas are malignant tumors arising from the fibrous tissue located just beneath the skin. They usually present as solitary, irregular masses on or protruding from the skin, especially in the flank, groin, and limb regions. Metastasis to the lungs and lymph nodes is not uncommon. Female cocker spaniels, boxers, and Boston terriers are at the highest risk of developing this type of cancer.

Diagnosis of fibrosarcoma is made through biopsy evaluation. Treatment involves a combination of surgery, radiation therapy, and cryotherapy.

Mast cell tumors (mastocytoma) may present as solitary or multiple skin nodules, some of which may be ulcerated and pigmented. Such tumors may be located anywhere on the dog, yet those hear the reproductive structures and on the digits of the feet seem to exhibit a higher degree of malignancy than those in other locations. These breeds are most commonly affected: boxers, Boston terriers, Labrador retrievers, bull terriers, dachshunds, and Weimaraners.

Mast cell tumors are especially significant because the cells making up the tumor are filled with granules containing histamine and several other powerful chemicals that can have profound effects on the body if released from the cells. Some of those effects are gastrointestinal ulcers, interference with normal blood clotting, and kidney inflammation.

Diagnosis of a mast cell tumor can often be made on cytological examination and biopsy of a tumor sample. In addition, evaluation of the blood often reveals abnormalities related to the release of histamine and other granules, such as low platelet counts, anemia, and elevations in white blood cells.

Because this neoplasia is stubborn, treatment for mast cell tumors employs a wide variety of techniques. Surgical excision of the visible mass along with a generous portion of the healthy tissue surrounding it (to ensure complete removal) is usually the first step. Veterinary surgeons must exercise extreme care when handling these tumors, since excessive handling could cause a massive release of granules from the tumor that can induce shock and collapse. Following surgical recovery, radiation therapy and chemotherapy may be employed to help reduce the chances of recurrence and metastatic growth. Cryotherapy is also employed when surgical excision of the tumor is incomplete or impossible.

Hemangiopericytomas are tumors arising from cells that line the blood vessels, especially those located in the limbs. They appear as isolated masses on the extremities that may be either soft or hard to the touch. Often, they are mistaken for lipomas. Ulceration of the tumor surface and secondary infections have been known to occur. Hemangiopericytomas are typically slow to metastasize.

Older female dogs have a higher incidence of this type of tumor than males. In addition, beagles, boxers, cocker spaniels, springer spaniels, and German shepherds are affected with greater frequency than other breeds.

Diagnosis of hemangiopericytomas is achieved through surgical biopsy. Complete surgical removal is the treatment of choice for these types of tumors. Because hemangiopericytomas have a high rate of recurrence, amputation of the affected leg may become necessary if tumor involvement is extensive. Radiation therapy is often used following surgical recovery to help reduce the chances of recurrence. Its effectiveness as a mode of therapy is highest in the early stages of tumor development.

Bladder tumors, relatively common in older dogs, can arise from the various tissues that make up this organ. The two most prevalent bladder neoplasms are transitional cell carcinoma and squamous cell carcinoma. Female dogs seem to be affected more often than males, and breed predispositions include Scottish terriers, beagles, collies, and Shetland sheepdogs.

Tumors within the urinary bladder can predispose to secondary infection and urolith formation. If the tumor is especially large, it can obstruct the outflow of urine and cause associated complications.

Clinical signs of a bladder tumor include bloody urine, stranguria, and painful urinations. Diagnosis is achieved through an evaluation of the urine as well as contrast radiographs or ultrasonography of the bladder. Biochemical evaluation of the blood may reveal elevated kidney enzymes if the kidneys have been damaged by obstruction of urine flow.

Both benign and malignant bladder tumors are best treated by surgical excision if their location and involvement permit. Unfortunately, most malignant bladder tumors are highly metastasizing; as a result, the chances of recurrence after surgery are high. For that reason, both chemotherapy and radiation therapy may be employed after surgery to help reduce the chances of recurrence and to attack any spread that may have taken place.

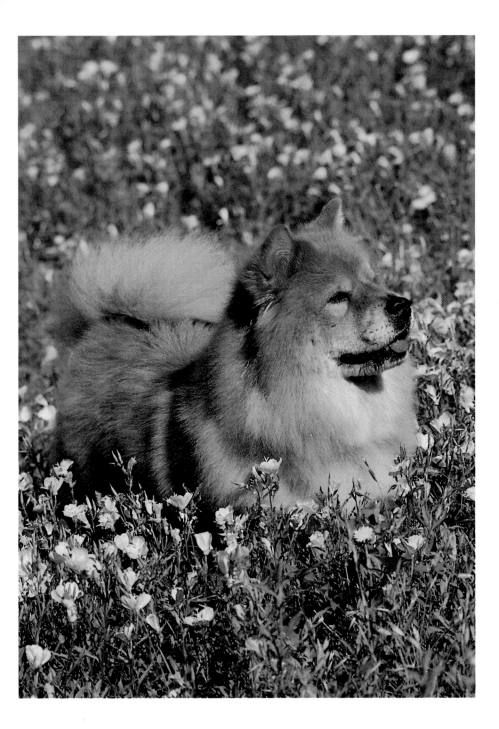

Chapter Five

Clinical Signs and Complaints

As your pet advances in years, you must become especially alert to changes in behavior or in physical anatomy and function that may signal the onset of disease. Your ability to distinguish actual disease conditions from normal age-related changes and to react accordingly is a critical key to extending your dog's life. Timing is of the essence when it comes to effective treatment or management of disease. The sooner a clinical sign is reported to your veterinarian, the better the chances are of identifying a disease and halting its progression.

Clinical signs (symptoms) are not disease entities in themselves, but rather the outward manifestations of disease. The onset of symptoms may occur acutely (suddenly) or slowly and progressively over a period of time. In some instances, the underlying disease condition causing the clinical sign may be in advanced development before the symptom appears. For example, pronounced weight loss, excessive thirst and urination, vomiting, and other signs linked to chronic kidney failure may not become readily apparent until at least 75 percent of the kidney tissue has been rendered nonfunctional. As a result, any delay in seeking professional help once symptoms appear could turn a manageable condition into a life-threatening crisis.

Please note that although the clinical signs and complaints presented in this section are among the more common encountered by owners of older dogs, they are not all-encompassing. In addition, the possible etiologies (causes) of each are certainly not limited to those listed. As a result, proper veterinary diagnosis of the actual underlying cause of your pet's clinical signs is essential.

Abdominal Pain

Abdominal pain in dogs is characterized by a tense abdomen that is noticeably tender to the touch. It usually has its origin in abnormal pressure within or stretching of an organ or organs, or in actual rupture of an organ. Dogs suffering from acute abdominal pain often exhibit a hunched, arched-back posture, with a reluctance to walk. Upon being handled, they may become aggressive because of pain. Depending upon the organ(s) involved, abdominal pain may also be accompanied by vomiting, diarrhea, icterus, seizures, abdominal swelling, and shock.

Diagnosis of the cause of abdominal pain is facilitated by a complete history and physical examination, blood profiles, and radiography or ultrasonography of the abdomen.

Immediate treatment for abdominal discomfort includes the use of

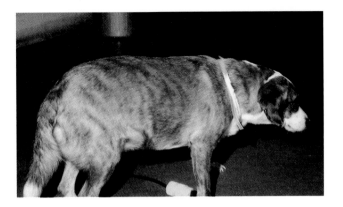

pain relievers or smooth muscle relaxants. In severe cases, intravenous fluid therapy and other supportive measures may be required, pending a diagnosis.

Abdominal pain.

Causes of Abdominal Pain in Older Dogs

Abdominal tumor
Bladder infection
Constipation
Gastric dilatation/volvulus
Gastroenteritis
Granuloma or abscess
Hepatitis
Intestinal foreign body and/or
  obstruction
Kidney disease
Organ rupture due to trauma or
  neoplasia
Pancreatitis
Prostate disease
Pyometra
Ulcers

Abdominal Swelling

Abdominal swelling may or may not be accompanied by abdominal pain. In most cases, noticeable swelling in older dogs is caused by fluid accumulation within the abdomen or by a bloated stomach. The onset of the clinical sign may provide clues to its origin. For instance, a sudden onset of abdominal swelling may be seen with bloat, internal hemorrhage, and organ rupture. Conversely, a slow, progressive onset is characteristic of congestive heart failure, neoplasia, and obesity. True abdominal swelling must be differentiated from the pot-bellied appearance caused by Cushing's disease or long-term steroid therapy in older dogs. That results not from internal disturbances within the

Causes of Abdominal Swelling in Older Dogs

Abdominal tumor
Ascites
Bladder distention
Constipation
Cushing's disease
Gastric dilatation/volvulus
Granuloma or abscess
Hemorrhage within the
  abdomen
Intestinal parasites
Liver disease
Obesity
Pregnancy

abdomen, but from thinning and sagging of the abdominal wall itself.

Apart from physical examination, identification of the cause of abdominal swelling is assisted by the use of radiographs. In addition, inserting a needle into the abdominal cavity and aspirating its contents, if any, can give a veterinarian

Causes of Polyphagia (Increased Appetite) in Older Dogs

Cushing's disease
Drug therapy (prednisolone)
Inadequate caloric intake
  (underfeeding)
Malabsorption/maldigestion of
  food
Intestinal parasitism

valuable insight into the cause. Treatment approaches are based upon diagnostic findings.

Appetite, Increased

A marked increase in appetite is termed polyphagia. Although the short-term health ramifications of polyphagia in dogs are not so significant as those of anorexia, its onset could indicate underlying disease and warrants due attention. In many instances, polyphagia can be induced when a dog is switched to a ration designed for seniors. Senior diets are lower in calories than those designed for young and middle-aged adults, and if portion sizes are not adjusted with the changeover, caloric deprivation and subsequent polyphagia can result. A multitude of diseases can also cause polyphagia. As a result, a veterinary evaluation is required if this symptom is seen. Once a diagnosis is achieved, treatment can be directed at correcting the underlying cause.

Appetite, Loss of

Anorexia is the medical term for loss of appetite. Although it is not unusual for a dog to go one or two days without eating, inappetence lasting three days or more should be considered abnormal. Left untreated, this reduction in caloric intake can lead to a state of starvation. That, in

Causes of Anorexia (Loss of Appetite) in Older Dogs

Addison's disease
Congestive heart failure
Dehydration
Dietary boredom
Fever
Gastrointestinal disease
Hypothyroidism
Kidney disease
Liver disease
Nausea
Pain
Pancreatitis

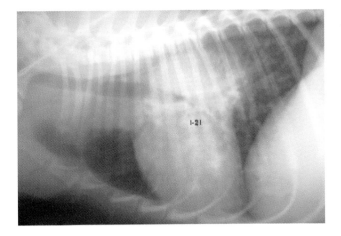

Mass located in the lungs, at the base of the heart, causing breathing difficulties.

turn, can lead to cachexia, diarrhea, anemia, poor wound healing, and immunosuppression.

Diagnosing the underlying cause of anorexia entails the use of behavioral history, physical examination, laboratory blood analysis, and, if needed, radiography. A lasting cure, of course, is dependent upon the underlying cause and its treatability. Special taste-tempting rations and medications, including B-vitamins and anabolic steroids, can be used to stimulate appetite.

Breathing Difficulties

Breathing difficulties in older dogs are usually the result of serious heart or lung disease or both. Respiratory distress may occur upon either the inhalation or the exhalation of air. Extreme care must be taken when handling distressed pets, since any degree of stress can lead to asphyxiation. Observation of breathing patterns, chest auscultation (with a stethoscope),

Causes of Breathing Difficulties in Older Dogs

Allergic bronchitis
Anemia
Chronic obstructive pulmonary disease
Heart disease and pulmonary edema
Heartworm disease
Obesity
Pleural effusions
Pneumonia
Pneumothorax
Respiratory foreign body
Respiratory neoplasia
Tracheal collapse
Tracheobronchitis

and chest radiographs are all useful in establishing a diagnosis. Often, nonspecific treatment must be initiated even before diagnostics can be performed. Such treatment would entail oxygen therapy, removal of any fluid accumulated in the chest with a needle and syringe or a drainage tube, and medications designed to dilate airways and blood vessels and move any fluid or edema out of the lungs. Once a diagnosis is achieved, specific treatment can be added.

Constipation

Constipation is a condition characterized by the inability to defecate with ease or regularity. It results in fecal retention within the colon. Tenesmus, or straining to defecate, usually accompanies constipation owing to the difficulty of passage. The dilemma tends to worsen over time, since the longer the feces is retained in the colon,

Impacted colon associated with constipation.

Causes of Constipation and Tenesmus in Older Dogs

Anal sac impaction/infection
Colon obstruction
Drug therapy
Enlarged prostate
Fluid imbalances
Foreign matter in stool
Fractured pelvis
Hypothyroidism
Intestinal parasites
Megacolon
Perineal hernia
Rectal polyps
Spinal cord trauma

the more moisture is reabsorbed by the colon, predisposing to even greater dryness and impaction. Other clinical signs of constipation include anxiousness, vocalizations while trying to eliminate, and a hunchbacked appearance. In severe, long-standing cases of constipation, loss of appetite, vomiting, and dehydration can be seen.

There are several potential causes of constipation in older pets. A definitive diagnosis of the underlying cause can generally be made through a history of the problem, physical examination, stool evaluations, and radiographs of the abdomen. Initial treatment for constipation involves emptying the colon by means of soapy, warm-water enemas. Sedation or anesthesia may be required for this proce-

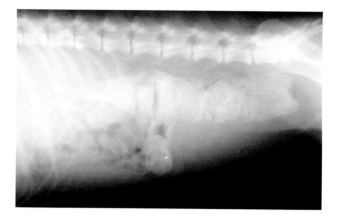

dure if the patient is in exceptional pain or excitable. For dogs under 20 pounds, 15 milliliters of warm, soapy water administered per rectum with a soft-tipped applicator or syringe will help soften the impacted stool. The procedure is repeated in 45 minutes if satisfactory results have not been obtained from the first enema. For senior canines weighing over 20 pounds, 25 to 40 milliliters per application usually does the trick. Commercially available enemas designed for human use are not suitable for dogs, since the contents of the enemas can cause severe dehydration and electrolyte imbalances.

In severe cases of constipation, intravenous fluid therapy may be required to restore water balance within the body and to help normalize large-intestinal function. Further, surgical intervention may be required in some instances to correct any underlying causes.

Long-term management procedures to prevent recurrence of constipation will depend upon the underlying cause of the disorder. Laxatives may be prescribed to help regulate the frequency of bowel movements. In addition, dietary adjustment, which can include increasing the amount of fiber in the ration, is an effective means of long-term management of constipation in older pets. Commercially available bran supplements or prescription dog foods containing higher amounts of fiber may be used to achieve that goal.

Coughing

Coughing is a reflex action initiated by stimulation of cough receptors located along the respiratory tract. Because the possible causes of coughing are so numerous, a step-by-step approach to diagnostics is often required to narrow the field of possible etiologies. Historical information and patient characteristics are important in establishing a diagnosis. For instance, heart disease and diseases of the trachea seem to affect smaller breeds more often than larger ones. Obesity can also predispose a dog to coughing from compression of fat on the respiratory tree. Further, by weakening the immune system, obesity can increase the susceptibility of the respiratory tract to infectious diseases and other conditions. Potential exposure to ill animals is also important in the differential diagnosis

Causes of Coughing in Older Dogs

Allergic bronchitis
Canine cough complex
Heart disease and pulmonary
  edema
Heartworm disease
Metastatic lung cancer
Pneumonia
Respiratory foreign body
Tonsillitis
Tracheal collapse
Tracheobronchitis

of coughing. For example, dogs that develop a cough following kenneling are likely to be suffering from infectious tracheobronchitis (canine cough).

The character of a cough is also important in establishing a diagnosis. For instance, dry, hacking coughs are characteristic of infectious tracheobronchitis, heartworm disease, and tumors of the lungs, whereas moist, productive coughs may be seen with heart disease and pneumonia. Coughing that occurs mainly at night often has a failing heart as its source, as do coughs that occur after strenuous exercise. Coughing that occurs after eating may signify a disease of the esophagus or mouth. Finally, buildup of respiratory secretions secondary to allergies or tonsillitis can cause a characteristic gagging cough (often mistaken for vomiting).

Tests and procedures utilized in the search for a diagnosis of a cough include a good history, physical examination, CBC, biochemistry profiles, chest and neck radiographs, heartworm testing, ultrasonography, endoscopy, and microscopic examination of sputum expelled during a coughing episode.

Treatment of coughing is dependent upon the underlying cause. Coughs of infectious origin are treated with antibiotics, nebulization therapy (inhalation of humidified or medicated air), and, if nonproductive in nature, cough suppressants. When a cough is productive, cough suppressants should not be used, since an accelerated buildup of respiratory secretions and inflammatory debris within the lungs would result. Finally, for coughs caused by heart disease, the use of appropriate therapy for that disorder should help resolve the cough.

Diarrhea

Diarrhea is a clinical sign of intestinal disease that is characterized by an abnormal increase in the water content of the feces, resulting in an increased frequency of elimination and volume of feces. Diarrhea marked by an abrupt, explosive onset—acute diarrhea—may be accompanied by lethargy, fever, or loss of appetite. Depending upon treatment, it usually runs its course within three to five days. Most cases of acute diarrhea, such as those caused by dietary indiscretions, are self-limiting; that is, they clear up on their own without specific treatment. However, cases persisting for more than 48 hours or accompanied by other clinical signs require veterinary evaluation. In those instances a specific diagnosis and treatment are needed to prevent dehydration, malnutrition, and, in severe cases, shock. Diarrhea that persists for more than 21 days or recurs on a periodic basis is deemed chronic. These chronic, or recurring, bouts can cause malnourishment and stress, both of which can suppress the immune system. Again, diagnosis of the

Causes of Diarrhea in Older Dogs

Addison's disease
Autoimmune disease
Bacterial intestinal infections
Dietary indiscretions/changes
Food allergy
Fungal infections
Intestinal foreign body
Intestinal neoplasia
Intestinal obstruction
Intestinal parasites
Kidney disease
Liver disease
Pancreatitis
Toxins/drugs
Viral intestinal infections

underlying cause and appropriate treatment are required.

As with vomiting, the potential causes of diarrhea in older dogs are diverse and abundant. A good history of the problem will help the veterinarian pinpoint the location of the disorder. For instance, if a dog is exhibiting elimination urgency because of the diarrhea, more than likely the diarrhea is originating in the large, rather than in the small, intestine. In addition, a black, tarry stool is usually indicative of small-intestinal bleeding and inflammation, whereas red blood in the stool occurs with large-intestinal inflammation. Potential exposure to other sick animals, foreign objects, or toxins is important information that can lead to a diagnosis.

The physical examination is another important tool for uncovering the source of diarrhea. For example, a dull, unthrifty hair coat could be indicative of a nutrient absorption disorder or internal parasites within the intestines. Further, pronounced weight loss could mean severe small-intestinal inflammation, liver or kidney disease, or even cancer. Finally, physical examination and abdominal palpation may detect obvious foreign bodies or masses involving the intestinal regions.

In addition to a physical exam, complete blood counts, serum biochemical profiles, urinalysis, fecal exams, radiography, ultrasonography, and endoscopy may be needed to achieve an exact diagnosis. Treatment of acute diarrhea with no other accompanying clinical signs consists of restricting food intake for a minimum of 24 hours. After this period, feeding may be resumed. Use a bland, low-fat diet for five to seven days (see Nutrition for Your Older Dog, p. 9). Bismuth subsalicylate mixtures available from grocery stores and pharmacies may also be administered at a dosage rate of one tablespoon or one tablet per 20 pounds every 12 hours to help treat diarrhea in older dogs.

For acute cases that fail to respond within 48 hours to the above treatments, or for those characterized by the presence of lethargy, fever, loss of appetite, or other clinical signs, veterinary intervention is required. Intravenous fluid therapy may be needed if the diarrhea has resulted in clinical dehydration. In addition to specific treatments aimed at the diagnosed cause, antidiarrheal medications designed to regulate fluid levels and motility within the intestines, anti-inflammatory medications, and intestinal surface protectants such as kaolin or bismuth may be prescribed.

Discharge: Nose, Eye, Ear, Reproductive

In veterinary medicine, drainage of fluid or semifluid material from an external opening or wound is termed a discharge. Discharges are responses to inflammation or build-up of fluid pressure within a tissue or organ space. The categories of discharges seen with greatest frequency in older dogs are nasal discharges, ocular (eye) discharges,

Nasal discharge.

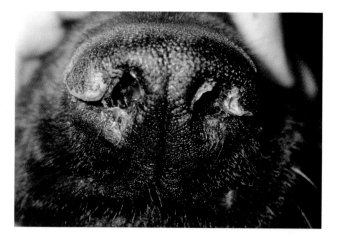

reproductive discharges, and ear discharges.

The color and character of a discharge can narrow the possibilities when it comes to identifying the cause. Serous discharges are thin, clear, and sometimes sticky. They are often seen in response to allergies, viral infections, and irritation from foreign matter. Mucoid discharges resemble mucus; they are often white to green in color, thick, and very stringy. They are sometimes seen in conjunction with or as a sequel to serous-type discharges, with the causes being very similar. Purulent discharges are characterized by the presence of pus. Very odorous, thick, and cream to green-brown in color, purulent discharges are seen whenever pus-producing bacterial infections are present. Those may be primary infections, or they may occur secondarily to other insults. In addition, fast-growing tumors causing extensive tissue damage can predispose to purulent-type discharges. Finally, sanguineous and hemorrhagic discharges have blood as a component (the latter type consisting almost entirely of blood) and are usually seen as a result of trauma, tumors, clotting disorders, poisonings, and certain infectious diseases. The discharges described above can exist independently or in combination with other types. For example, a discharge that contains both mucus and pus is called a mucopurulent discharge. Similarly, a serous discharge that is blood-

Causes of Discharges in Older Dogs

Discharges involving the ears
Bacterial infection (purulent, hemorrhagic)
Trauma (hemorrhagic)
Yeast infection (brown, odorous)

Discharges involving the eyes
Allergies (serous, mucoid)
Bacterial infection (purulent)
Foreign matter (serous, mucoid)
Keratoconjunctivitis sicca (mucoid, purulent)
Neoplasia/cyst (mucoid, purulent, hemorrhagic)
Trauma (hemorrhagic, serous)
Viral infection (serous)

Discharges involving the nose
Allergies (serous, mucoid)
Bacterial infection (purulent, sanguineous)
Blood clotting disorder (hemorrhagic)
Foreign body (serous, mucoid, purulent, hemorrhagic)
Fungal infection (purulent, sanguineous, hemorrhagic)
Open socket due to tooth loss (purulent, hemorrhagic)
Periodontal disease (purulent, hemorrhagic)
Trauma (hemorrhagic)
Tumor, polyp (purulent, sanguineous, hemorrhagic)
Viral infection (serous, sanguineous)

Discharges involving the reproductive tract
Bacterial infection (purulent, hemorrhagic)
Neoplasia/cyst (mucoid, purulent, hemorrhagic)
Prostatitis (purulent, hemorrhagic)
Tumor, polyp (purulent, sanguineous, hemorrhagic)
Vaginitis/metritis (purulent, hemorrhagic)

tinged is referred to as a serosanguineous discharge.

Diagnosis of the underlying cause of a discharge will involve analysis of historical complaints of the problem, a complete physical examination, and appropriate laboratory tests. Often, microscopic examination of the discharge leads a veterinarian to a diagnosis with no further laboratory workup required. In difficult cases, however, radiographs or endoscopic examina-

tions may be necessary to pinpoint the exact etiology.

Treatment for a discharge will be geared to correcting the underlying cause. For instance, serous nasal discharges caused by allergies often respond to nasal decongestants and anti-inflammatory medications. Purulent discharges signify the need for appropriate antibiotic therapy to bring the infection under control. Hemorrhagic discharges from the vagina of an intact female

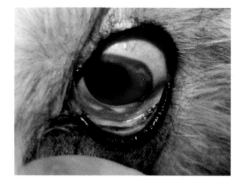

dog over eight years of age usually warrant an ovariohysterectomy. Discharges from the ears are usually caused by infectious agents or parasites and need to be treated accordingly. Finally, mucoid discharges from the eyes may necessitate the need for artificial tear or cyclosporine application on a daily basis (see KCS, p. 109).

Ear, Deafness In

See The Ears, p. 112.

Eye, Blindness In

See The Eyes, p. 107.

Eye, Redness or Cloudiness of

Inflammation involving the conjunctival membrane lining the eye socket and the sclera (the white portion of the eyeball) creates the appearance of a "red eye" in dogs.

Inflammation usually is accompanied by squinting (photophobia) and a discharge, either clear or mucoid. Clear discharges are usually indicative of allergies and surface irritations; thicker mucoid discharges accompany actual infections, foreign bodies, and keratoconjunctivitis sicca. Apart from cataracts and age-related sclerosis of the lens, a cloudy appearance may result from edema, scarring, or pigmentation of the cornea secondary to inflammation, corneal ulceration, keratoconjunctivitis sicca, or increases in intraocular pressures.

Careful ophthalmologic examinations, followed by special tests to check the pressure within the affected eye(s) and tear production, usually lead to a diagnosis. As always, treatment will be geared to the underlying cause. If foreign body

Causes of Eye Redness or Cloudiness in Older Dogs

Allergies
Bacterial infection
Cataracts
Corneal pigmentation
Foreign matter
Fungal infection (blastomycosis, histoplasmosis, cryptococcosis)
Glaucoma
Keratoconjunctivitis sicca
Lenticular sclerosis (cloudiness)
Neoplasia/cyst
Trauma
Viral infection

irritation is suspected, flushing the eye thoroughly with warm water will be of some benefit. If the corneal surface of the eye is not ulcerated, anti-inflammatory ointments and drops can be used to reduce inflammation and redness, while antibiotics are indicated in cases of infection and corneal ulcers. (For specific treatments for glaucoma, KCS, and cataracts, see The Eyes, p. 107.)

Facial Features, Drooping of

See Paralysis, p. 146.

Facial Swelling

Facial swelling can have a number of etiologies in older dogs. The nature and location of the swelling are important for diagnostic purposes. For instance, semifirm to fluctuant localized swellings that are painful to the touch are likely to be abscesses, salivary mucocoeles, or sites of bite or sting wounds. Localized swellings that are firm or hard to the touch are usually caused by tumors, chronic infections, or enlarged lymph nodes. Diffuse, symmetrical swellings can most often be attributed to allergic reactions. Regardless of the cause, swellings involving the facial regions should be attended to promptly. Though most are associated only with pain and discomfort, some can become life-threatening if their development

Causes of Facial Swelling in Older Dogs

Allergic reaction to insect sting
Fever
Jaw fracture
Lymphatic obstruction
Oral foreign body
Oral or bone tumor
Salivary cyst
Snake bite
Tooth abscess

impedes the normal flow of air through the nose or trachea.

The first step in obtaining a definitive diagnosis of facial swelling is to inquire into potential exposure to snakes, insects, or aggressive animals. A thorough physical exam is also warranted, along with cytology of the swelling. Radiographs are useful in select instances as well. Treatment is based upon diagnostic findings. In allergic reactions, a combination of antihistamine and anti-inflammatory injections will alleviate an acute swelling quite effectively.

Fever

The normal temperature range for a dog is 99.5°F to 102.8°F. Any elevation of temperature above the latter figure in the absence of previous exercise or rigorous activity should be considered abnormal. Dogs exhibiting elevated temperatures usually show signs of lethargy,

Causes of True Fever in Older Dogs

Autoimmune disease
Drug therapy
Infection
Inflammation due to disease or injury
Neoplasia

Causes of Hyperthermia in Older Dogs

Excitement/fear
Heat stroke
Overexertion
Seizures

inappetence, and malaise. Other indications of fever in dogs include shivering, piloerection (hair standing on end), curling up, and an active search for warmth.

It is important to differentiate true fever from hyperthermia. Both conditions are characterized by elevated body temperatures, but their causes are very different. True fever occurs when the body readjusts its "thermostat" in the brain in response to inflammation, infection, or the release of certain chemicals. In cases of true fever, body temperature rarely exceeds 107°F. In contrast, hyperthermia results from the body's being subjected to excessive muscular exertion or external heat sources. For instance, increased muscle activity associated with seizures in older dogs can quickly lead to a hyperthermic state. Heat stroke, a severe form of hyperthermia, occurs in dogs exposed to high environmental temperatures. In some cases of heat stroke, body temperatures can rise beyond 110°F. Obviously, such a condition will lead to death if not recognized and treated promptly.

To obtain your dog's temperature, insert a plastic digital thermometer into its rectum for one to two minutes. Glass thermometers should not be used because of the danger of breakage. Although any elevation in temperature is significant, temperatures exceeding 105°F should be considered medical emergencies; they warrant immediate attention.

Treatment of true fever is geared to treating the underlying cause, once diagnosed. Anti-inflammatory medications designed to reduce the fever may be administered while the diagnostic workup is being performed. Aspirin and acetaminophen can both be effective for that purpose. The dosage of aspirin, given orally every 8 hours, generally should not exceed 15 mg per pound of body weight. The dose of acetaminophen, given orally every 12 hours, should not exceed 5 mg per pound of body weight. Before giving any medication, check with your veterinarian to confirm the exact dosage for your particular pet. Note: Ibuprofen should never be given to a dog unless specifically prescribed by a veterinarian.

If hyperthermia is diagnosed or even suspected, whole body cooling is the only effective method of reducing body temperature. Immersing affected dogs in ice water baths or administering alcohol baths will help rapidly lower body temperatures to safe levels. Cold water enemas may be given to expedite the process. These procedures should be continued until a body temperature of 103°F is achieved. Once that is accomplished, cooling procedures should be discontinued to prevent accidental hypothermia.

Incoordination, Falling, and Circling

Incoordination, falling, and circling are usually caused by disorders affecting the nervous system. The onset of these activities may be either sudden or progressive, and they may appear in conjunction. Falling and incoordination must be differentiated from true weakness, which can have an entirely different set of causes (see Weakness, p. 155). The former result from a deficiency in proprioception, which is the nervous system's ability to coordinate limb, eye, and body movements with sensory input. Circling is usually caused by inflammation or direct pressure placed upon the brain.

Care must be taken when interacting with pets exhibiting any of these clinical signs, since disorientation could lead to sudden aggressiveness. Diagnostic efforts should be directed at the brain, spinal cord,

Causes of Incoordination, Falling, and Circling in Older Dogs

---

Ear infection
Fracture
Infection involving nervous
  system
Inflammation of brain or spinal
  cord
Intervertebral disk disease
Poisoning
Trauma involving nervous
  system
Vestibular disease

or ears. Nonspecific treatments for incoordination, falling, and circling include strict confinement to prevent self-injury, sedatives, and anti-inflammatory medications, pending a definitive diagnosis.

Jaundice (Icterus)

Jaundice, or icterus, is a clinical sign characterized by a yellow-orange discoloration of, among

Causes of Jaundice in Older Dogs

Bile duct obstruction
Gall bladder disease
Internal bleeding and/or
  destruction of red blood cells
Liver disease

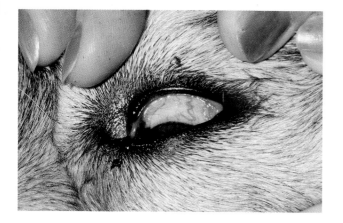

Jaundice: Note the yellow tint to the sclera of the eye.

other things, the skin and mucous membranes. It is the result of elevated levels of bile pigments in the bloodstream. It represents serious clinical disease and warrants prompt diagnosis and treatment of the underlying cause.

Lameness

Lameness is defined as the inability or reluctance to bear complete weight on one or more limbs. There are various degrees of lameness, the severity of which can help lead to a diagnosis. For instance, lameness in which the pet refuses to bear weight on the affected limb is usually indicative of a bone fracture or a joint dislocation. Older dogs affected with a non-weight-bearing lameness usually carry the affected limb close to the body, with all joints flexed. Lameness that involves only a partial loss in function, sometimes referred to as a limp, can be caused by minor fractures and a multitude of

other conditions, most of which are listed below.

A thorough history of the lameness will expedite the diagnostic process. It should include answers to these questions: When was the lameness first noticed? What time of day is the lameness most noticeable? Did it have a sudden or a progressive onset? Has the pet experienced any trauma within the past four to six weeks? Have there been other changes in activity or behavior along with the lameness? In addition a thorough veterinary orthopedic examination should be per-

Causes of Lameness in Older Dogs

Arthritis
Bruised or traumatized foot pad
Degenerative joint disease
Foreign body penetration
Fracture
Fungal disease
Hip dislocation
Hypothyroidism and other
 metabolic diseases
Infections involving
 bones/joints/muscles
Intervertebral disk disease
Joint sprain or strain
Lyme disease
Metabolic bone disease
Muscle trauma/bruising
Myopathy/myelopathy
Neoplasia
Patellar luxation

formed. During that examination, a veterinarian should be able to ascertain the exact location of the lameness, its extent, and possibly its cause. For example, swelling, bruising, and pain at any point along a bone or joint often indicate that a fracture or ligament tear is present. Hard masses beneath the skin overlying or involving a bone or joint may lead a clinician to suspect a tumor or a chronic infection. Several types of fungal diseases, such as blastomycosis, histoplasmosis, coccidioidomycosis, and cryptococcosis, can cause prominent and painful bone and joint swellings that are often accompanied by clinical signs of disease related to other organ systems, including the skin, eyes, nervous system, and respiratory system. Finally, degenerative joint diseases, especially those involving the hip joints, can lead to a noticeable loss in muscle mass in the hip and thigh regions that is often diagnostic.

Such histories and physical examination findings can lead to a tentative diagnosis of the etiology of a lameness. However, radiographs, joint fluid analysis, biopsy procedures, and other laboratory tests may be needed to make a tentative diagnosis definitive.

Treatment for lameness will depend upon the definitive diagnosis. For minor ligament sprains and muscle strains, as well as arthritic flare-ups, three to five days of forced rest, in combination with the administration of anti-inflammatory pain relievers such as buffered aspirin, will help to resolve minor lameness. Other etiologies will need to be addressed with medications and corrective procedures specific to the condition in question.

Odors: Body, Breath

Noxious odors associated with older dogs usually result from disease conditions that require veterinary attention. Careful examination of the oral cavity, skin, and hair coat will often reveal the source of the problem. In some cases, more diagnostics may be required. If the underlying condition is properly

Causes of Noxious Odors in Older Dogs

Breath
Anal sac disease
Coprophagy
Kidney disease
Oral foreign body
Oral ulcer
Periodontal disease
Tumors of the oral cavity

Skin, Hair Coat, General
Colitis
Ear infections
External sources—skunks, feces, and the like
Seborrhea
Skin infections
Skin tumors

diagnosed and treated, the unpleasant odor usually can be lessened or eliminated.

Paralysis

Paralysis affecting older dogs can be divided into two types: sensory paralysis and motor paralysis. Sensory paralysis is characterized by loss of touch and pain sensation in the affected portions of the body. This type of paralysis is serious, since it can predispose to self-mutilation. In canines, sensory paralysis is usually accompanied by flaccid motor paralysis, a condition in which the muscles responsible for movement fail to receive nervous impulses and are therefore rendered nonfunctional. In contrast, spastic motor paralysis is charac-

terized by muscular rigidity and spasticity caused by uncontrolled and continuous nervous impulses to the muscles. With such a paralysis, the limbs and neck assume extended rigid positions that make locomotion impossible. Spastic motor paralysis is most commonly seen with malicious poisonings.

Paralysis may also affect certain internal organs if the nerves innervating those organs are disrupted or damaged. For instance, paralysis of the bladder or colon will result in the overaccumulation of wastes in those organs. In addition, paralysis can play a role in the development of the condition of the esophagus known as megaesophagus, characterized by a flaccid esophagus that is unable to contract and expel food into the stomach. As foodstuffs accumulate within the paralyzed organ, the dog becomes more prone to regurgitation and asperation pneumonia, the latter of which can become life threatening.

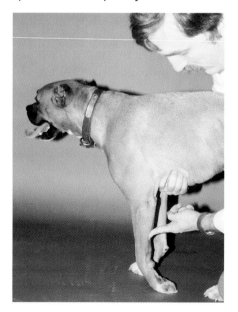

Paralysis affecting the forelimb of a dog.

Diagnosing the specific cause of paralysis requires a good history (including potential exposure to poisons), physical examination, and other diagnostic tests deemed necessary, including those specific to nervous system maladies. Treatment will be determined by the underlying cause. Drugs to reduce inflammation are indicated if intervertebral disk disease, trauma, or other inflammatory disorders are diagnosed. In addition, muscle relaxants may be indicated in cases of spastic paralysis. Finally, when sensory paralysis has affected a limb, amputation may be required to prevent self-mutilation and subsequent gangrene.

Regurgitation

See Vomiting, p. 154.

Salivation, Excessive

Excessive salivation, or drooling, is a clinical sign of disease affecting either the oral cavity, esophagus, or stomach. It may also be secondary to seizures and other neurological illnesses. Diagnosis of an underlying cause begins with careful examination of the oral cavity for any obvious abnormalities. Then, the veterinarian may proceed with specific testing procedures aimed at identifying other potential etiologies. As always,

Causes of Excessive Salivation in Older Dogs

Esophageal obstructions
Foreign body within oral cavity
Jaw fractures
Nausea
Oral mass or tumor
Periodontal disease
Poisoning
Rabies (rare)
Reactions to noxious objects or
 chemicals
Seizures

treatment will be customized to the diagnosis. In the case of excessive salivation caused by the consumption of medications, plants, insects, or other irritants, rinsing the mouth with copious amounts of water will to dilute the noxious substance and diminish this clinical sign. If a foreign object is lodged between the teeth or in the gums, tweezers can be used to extract the object, if the patient allows.

Seizures

A seizure is defined as uncontrollable behavior or muscle activity caused by an abnormal increase in nervous system activity. Seizures in older dogs can occur to varying degrees. Although when we think of a seizure we usually envision a full-blown convulsion, seizures should be suspected whenever a

Causes of Seizures in Older Dogs

Brain inflammation secondary
  to trauma
Brain tumor
Heat stroke
Idiopathic epilepsy
Kidney disease
Liver disease
Low blood sugar
Poisoning

dog exhibits unusual or unexplained behavioral changes.

Depending upon the underlying cause, seizures can be continuous and unrelenting, as seen in certain types of poisonings, or sporadic and of short duration, as in many cases of true epilepsy. The duration of the actual seizure episode is directly proportional to its danger. Typically, seizure episodes lasting over three minutes should be regarded as medical emergencies warranting prompt veterinary attention.

In older dogs, seizure activity must be differentiated from syncope, a loss of consciousness caused by oxygen deprivation to the brain. The two most common causes of syncope in mature canines are heart failure and anemia. An older dog may appear fine one moment, then suddenly collapse and lose consciousness as a result of oxygen deficiency. Such an episode is often mistaken for a seizure.

The typical epileptic seizure has three distinct phases. The first, called the preictal phase, is characterized by anxiety and restlessness. The ictal phase, or true seizure, follows it. Recumbency, uncontrolled muscular contractions and eye movements, and spontaneous urination or defecation are seen during this phase. The postictal phase following the true seizure is characterized by staggering, depression, confusion, and exhaustion. It usually lasts from 15 minutes to six hours.

As with other symptoms, diagnosis of the cause of a seizure is based upon analysis of the characteristics and frequency of the seizure activity, a physical examination, and appropriate laboratory tests, including a complete blood profile and urinalysis. If no underlying cause can be pinpointed for recurring seizures, a tentative diagnosis of idiopathic epilepsy is usually made. Idiopathic epilepsy can show up at any age, and it may last only a short while before disappearing for good.

To prevent seizures from recurring, treatment must be geared to correcting the underlying cause. When a cause cannot be discovered, or when the underlying disease is incurable, anticonvulsant medications such as primidone or phenobarbital and its derivatives may be necessary to control seizure activity. Initially, frequent adjustments to the dosages of these medications may be necessary, in an attempt to discover the ideal dose that will control seizures, yet cause minimal depression in the patient. In addition, because anticonvulsant medications can place undue stress on the liver, older dogs receiving such drugs should have a liver function test at least once a year.

If your dog suffers a seizure, do not attempt to intervene or hold your pet down during the ictal phase. That could cause injury to your dog as well as to yourself. Instead, throw a thick blanket or towel over your dog and wait out the seizure. Then confine your dog to a small bathroom or travel kennel until the disorientation associated with the postictal phase has disappeared. If the ictal phase has extended beyond three minutes, wrap your pet securely in the blanket, taking care not to be bitten, and transport it in this way to your veterinarian.

Skin, Dry and Flaky

See Seborrhea, p. 102.

Skin: Hair Loss (Alopecia) and Itching

Hair loss due to the presence of disease may be differentiated from hair loss due to normal shedding by the appearance of bald patches of skin. In older dogs, alopecia may occur secondary to inflammation or changes within hair follicles caused by underlying disease, or to relentless chewing and scratching by the dog itself.

Causes of Hair Loss or Itching in Older Dogs

Allergies
Bacterial skin infections
Chronic illness
Cushing's disease
Diabetes mellitus
Hypothyroidism
Nutritional deficiency
Seborrhea
Self-trauma
Skin parasites (fleas, mites, ringworm)
Stress

The distribution of the hair loss can provide valuable clues to the underlying cause. For example, alopecia that is symmetrical (affecting both sides of the body equally) is usually caused by disturbances originating within the body, including allergies, nutritional deficiencies, and endocrine maladies. In contrast, patchy, random hair loss is usually seen with infections or

Hair loss may be associated with itching.

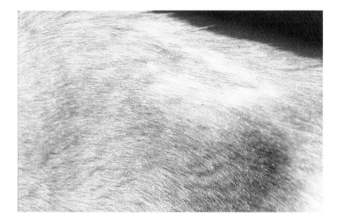

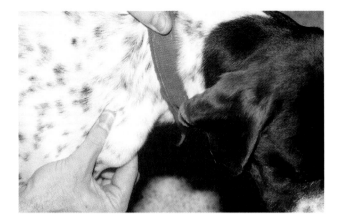

ing and encourage hair regrowth. Daily brushing also stimulates hair growth and replacement while helping to soothe itchy skin.

Skin: Lumps and Masses on or Beneath

A mass or lump on or beneath the skin of an older dog warrants prompt veterinary attention. Certainly the first thought that comes to mind is cancer, yet that is not always the diagnosis. There are several conditions that may appear to be neoplasia, yet are entirely different in origin. Granulomas represent a type of immune response by the dog's body to a foreign body, fungi, or certain types of bacteria. Consisting of an accumulation of inflammatory cells, granulomas are well defined, symmetrical, and self-limiting as far as their growth is concerned. Cysts are fluid- or debris-filled sacs that may arise spontaneously or in con-

parasites. The presence or absence of itching along with the alopecia is also significant in determining a diagnosis. Itching results from inflammation within the skin or the hair follicles, and it is usually seen along with hair loss. However, hair loss can also occur in the absence of itching. In such instances, the underlying cause is a hormonal imbalance, nutritional disorder, stress, ringworm (a fungal infection), or demodex mange.

Once a diagnosis has been established, treatment of the underlying disorder will reverse most cases of alopecia. However, hair regrowth may be slow or may not occur at all if scarring has taken place within the skin and hair follicles or if the underlying disease condition cannot be medically managed.

Anti-inflammatory medications, special diets, antihistamines plus fatty acid supplements (see Allergies, p. 99), medicated shampoos, and topical moisturizing sprays may all be prescribed to discourage itch-

Causes of Lumps or Masses on or beneath the Skin

Abscess
Cyst
Fibrous nodular scar
Granuloma
Swollen lymph node(s)
Tumor, benign or malignant

junction with other diseases. The most prevalent type of cyst in older dogs is the sebaceous cyst, a firm, nodular structure that may be felt just beneath the skin. Sebaceous cysts result from the accumulation and hardening of oily sebum within sebaceous glands located in the skin. True abscesses are caused by localized regions of bacterial infection. Soft, fluctuant, and painful when touched, abscesses are usually accompanied by fever and some degree of malaise. Finally, fibrous nodular scarring can occur secondary to foreign body penetration or most commonly, following vaccine administrations. Usually no bigger than marbles, these nodules, with time, usually regress on their own.

Identification of a mass or lump can be made through the use of cytology. If neoplasia is suspected, an actual biopsy will be required as well. The primary treatment for the majority of lumps or masses on or beneath the skin is surgical excision. In the case of abscesses, surgical drainage along with appropriate antibiotic therapy will be required for resolution.

Sneezing

Sneezing is a reflex act that is initiated by irritation within a portion of the respiratory system, namely the nasal cavity and surrounding tissues. A nasal discharge may accompany sneezing episodes. To

Causes of Sneezing in Older Dogs

Allergic rhinitis
Infection of nasal passages and/or sinuses
Nasal foreign body
Nasal polyp or tumor

identify the underlying etiology of the sneezing, a number of procedures are used. Apart from a standard physical examination and blood analysis, direct visual examination of the nasal passages while a pet is under sedation is the most valuable tool in the diagnostic process. At that time, samples of nasal secretions may be obtained for microscopic review, and radiographs of the nasal passages may be taken if necessary.

Sneezing caused by an infection within the nasal passages may be managed through the use of appropriate antimicrobial medications. Tumors and polyps involving the nasal passages are often treated with surgery or radiation to help achieve remission while alleviating the sneezing. In cases of sneezing caused by allergies, antihistamines and anti-inflammatory medications are usually effective in controlling clinical signs.

Thirst, Excessive

See Urination, Excessive, p. 152.

**Causes of Increased
Thirst/Excessive Urination
in Older Dogs**

Addison's disease
Bladder infection
Cushing's disease
Diabetes insipidus
Diabetes mellitus
Drug therapy (corticosteroids)
Increase in physical activity
Kidney disease
Liver disease
Mineral/electrolyte imbalances
Poisoning
Prostate disease
Stress
Uterine infection (pyometra)

Urination, Excessive

Polyuria/polydipsia(PU/PD) is defined as an abnormal elevation in urine output (PU) and an abnormal increase in water consumption (PD). PU\PD is a fairly common complaint in older pets. Polyuria must be differentiated from another condition that often affects older dogs: urinary incontinence. Since the underlying causes and health ramifications of these two conditions can be very different from one another, a thorough diagnostic workup is warranted. Normal daily urine output for a dog should not exceed 40 milliliters per kilogram of body weight. Output greater than that, as measured by a veterinarian, is considered polyuria. Special laboratory tests of urine samples and blood serum can determine the filtration rate of the kidneys and their ability to conserve water within the body, thereby providing a definitive diagnosis. Of course, once polyuria/polydipsia is determined, the underlying cause must be uncovered before effective treatment can be applied.

Urination: Incontinence

Urinary incontinence is a clinical sign associated with diseases affecting the urinary system and the nervous system. It is characterized by the inability of a dog to control the flow of urine from the bladder. Incontinence may appear as a sudden, unexpected flow of urine or as a continuous urine drip. In older dogs, its occurrence is often limited to the nighttime hours. Dogs that are incontinent usually experience irritation and inflammation of the external genitalia and surrounding skin because of urine scalding.

**Potential Causes of Urinary
Incontinence in Older Dogs**

Idiopathic (of unknown cause)
Spinal cord injury/disease
Urethral obstruction
Urinary tract infection
Urinary uroliths

Because the potential causes of incontinence are so numerous, diagnosis of the underlying source can be difficult. Tests that focus on both the urinary and the nervous systems will be needed. As with other symptoms, treatment of urinary incontinence will depend upon its cause. For older, spayed female dogs suffering from idiopathic (of unknown origin) incontinence, newer medications now available can increase sphincter tone within the lower portion of the urinary tract and help curb incontinence.

Urination: Straining (Stranguria)

Apparent difficulty in voiding urine is a clinical sign of lower urinary tract disease. Overdistention of the bladder wall by urine stimulates an abnormal urge to urinate, as do irritation and inflammation affecting the bladder and urethral linings. Bloody urine in dogs straining to urinate is either due to the underlying disease or secondary to the excessive straining itself. Oftentimes, crystals that have formed within the urine nick and cut the inner surfaces of the bladder and urethra and create an intense urge to urinate, even when no urine is produced.

When a dog exhibits stranguria, the veterinarian has to determine whether the bladder is full or empty. Stranguria accompanied by an empty bladder often signifies

Causes of Stranguria in Older Dogs

Neoplasia
Prostate enlargement
Spinal nerve damage
Trauma to bladder or urethra
Urinary infection
Urinary uroliths

inflammation, in the absence of an obstruction. In these instances, treatment of the underlying cause and use of smooth-muscle relaxants can provide relief to a distressed pet. However, dogs that exhibit stranguria yet have a full bladder may be suffering from an obstruction. If an obstruction is indeed causing the bladder to overfill, the stranguria will be accompanied by a painful abdomen and intense restlessness. Prompt urinary catheterization is needed to restore urine flow. If that is not performed kidney failure, bladder rupture, or death could result.

Uroliths removed from the bladder of an older dog exhibiting stranguria (straining to urinate).

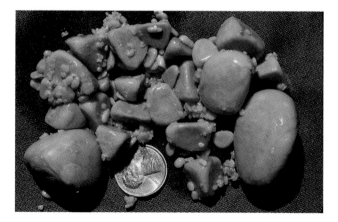

Vomiting

Vomiting is the forceful expulsion of stomach contents through the mouth. This act must be differentiated from regurgitation, which is the passive expulsion of food from the esophagus, not the stomach. Regurgitation is caused by disorders involving the esophagus, including esophagitis and megaesophagus.

Vomiting is a reflex act resulting from stimulation of receptors in the brain and various organs throughout the body. Stimulation of those receptors can result from inflammation, irritation, distension, pressure, or toxins. Multiple vomiting episodes are usually indicative of a serious underlying disorder, and they can quickly lead to electrolyte imbalances, dehydration, and shock. As a result, an underlying cause must be identified as rapidly as possible so that proper treatment can be instituted. Vaccination history, parasite prevention, and potential exposure to sick animals, toxins, drugs, or foreign bodies are all important pieces of information that can lead to a diagnosis. In most cases, a thorough physical examination and a laboratory work-up are needed to uncover the exact cause of the vomiting and any secondary complications, such as dehydration. Examples of appropriate laboratory work include complete blood counts, serum biochemical evaluations, fecal examination for internal parasites, radiographs (including contrast studies using barium swallows), and endoscopy. Exploratory surgery may also be required if the above measures fail to yield a diagnosis.

Specific treatment of a vomiting dog is dependent upon the underlying cause. For uncomplicated cases in which vomiting occurs no more than twice, withholding food and water for at least 24 hours often allows the body to recover on its own. However, if multiple episodes occur, vigorous treatment is required, including intravenous

Causes of Vomiting in Older Dogs

Addison's disease
Bacterial gastrointestinal
  infections
Brain disorders
Diabetes mellitus
Dietary indiscretions/changes
Food allergies
Gastric dilatation/Volvulus
Gastric ulcers
Gastrointestinal neoplasia
Gastrointestinal obstruction
Inflammatory bowel disease
Ingestion of a foreign body
Intestinal parasites
Kidney disease
Liver disease
Pyometra
Stress
Toxins/Drugs
Vestibular disorders
Viral gastrointestinal infections

fluid therapy to correct or prevent dehydration and electrolyte imbalances. Antivomiting medications, as well as antibiotics to control secondary infections, may be necessary also.

Weakness

Weakness as a clinical sign can arise from disorders involving a number of body systems, including the circulatory, respiratory, nervous, musculoskeletal, and endocrine systems. Episodes of weakness are often shrugged off as a normal consequence of aging or arthritis, when in reality a serious medical condition may be the source. The intensity of these bouts of weakness can range from moderate lethargy to actual collapse. The duration of the episodes often can provide valuable clues to the underlying etiology. For instance, episodes lasting less than one minute are usually related to heart and lung disease. Incidents lasting over one minute but less than five can often be attributed to seizure activity. Persistent, continuous weakness can result from neurological, endocrine, or musculoskeletal disorders, not to mention severe heart disease and anemia.

Since weakness is a nonspecific sign with a host of potential causes, a careful step-by-step approach to diagnostics is indicated. Starting with a thorough history and physical exam, diagnostic protocol may

Causes of Weakness in Older Dogs

Anemia
Arthritis
Heart disease
Heartworm disease
Hypothyroidism
Intervertebral disk disease
Kidney disease
Low blood glucose
Lung disease
Myelopathy
Myopathy
Neoplasia
Neuropathy
Poisoning
Spondylosis deformans

extend to laboratory testing of the blood, urine, and stool, ECGs, radiographs, ultrasound, and a variety of other specialized tests. Once a cause is uncovered, appropriate treatment may be administered.

Weight Loss (Cachexia)

In dogs, a progressive loss of body weight in the absence of a predetermined weight loss program could signify the presence of an underlying disease. The term cachexia is used to describe weight loss and wasting occurring secondary to disease. The potential causes of cachexia in older dogs

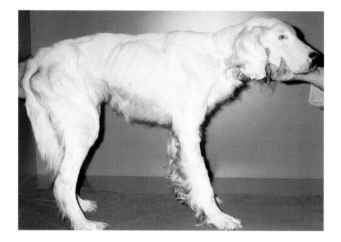

Causes of Cachexia (Weight Loss) in Older Dogs

Chronic infections
Diabetes mellitus
Gastrointestinal parasites
Heart disease
Hypoadrenocorticism
Kidney disease
Liver disease
Maldigestion of food
Neoplasia
Starvation

A severe case of cachexia.

are numerous. A thorough medical history, physical examination, laboratory workup, and radiographs can all be utilized to pinpoint the cause of the problem.

Once a proper diagnosis has been made, specific treatment can be undertaken to cure or manage the underlying disorder. In addition, high-energy diets, food supplements, anabolic steroids, and exercise may all be prescribed to help reverse a pet's cachexic state.

Chapter Six

Select First Aid Procedures for Older Dogs

As your dog grows older, you are more likely to be faced with an emergency created by injury or illness. If you suddenly find yourself in such a situation, don't panic! Remember that the purpose of any type of first aid is to stabilize your pet until veterinary care can be obtained. Begin by ascertaining whether the situation is life-threatening. Cessation of breathing, loss of pulse or heartbeat, extensive bleeding and trauma, and poisoning are life-threatening circumstances that warrant the prompt rendering of first aid.

Always use caution when interacting with injured or ill dogs; they may exhibit aggressiveness if in pain or distress. If need be, muzzle your pet with a piece of gauze, belt, leash or necktie before you handle it. However, do not apply a muzzle if your pet is vomiting or having breathing difficulties; instead, use a thick blanket or heavy-duty gloves when handling or transporting your dog if it exhibits aggressiveness.

Once first aid has been initiated, transport your pet to the veterinarian as soon as possible. Be sure to call the veterinary office beforehand to describe your pet's condition and give your estimated time of arrival. That will enable the staff to provide swift emergency care upon your arrival. Note: If you suspect that your dog has suffered a neck or spinal injury, transport it on a board or window screen to keep from aggravating the injury.

Artificial Respiration

Artificial respiration should be performed if your pet has stopped breathing. To determine whether that has occurred, observe the chest for breathing movements or hold a mirror in front of your pet's nose. If it is breathing, condensation should be visible on the mirror surface. If your dog is not breathing:

Table 13:
Normal Physiologic Values for Dogs

Temperature (degrees Fahrenheit)	99.5–102.8
Pulse (beats per minute)	60–120
Respirations (per minute)	14–22

- Determine whether a heartbeat or pulse is present. If not, be prepared to integrate external heart massage with artificial respiration.
- Clear the mouth of any vomitus, blood, debris, or foreign objects. Pull the tongue straight out, then close the dog's mouth.
- Place your mouth over your pet's nose and blow air into the nostrils until you see the chest expand.
- Release the seal and allow the dog to exhale.
- Repeat this sequence every five seconds until your dog is breathing on its own or until veterinary care is obtained.

External Heart Massage

If no heartbeat or pulse can be seen, felt, or heard, external heart massage must be initiated in conjunction with artificial respiration. First perform an artificial respiration, and then:

- Position your dog on its right side.
- Place the heel of one hand on the front third of the ribcage just behind the elbow, then place the other hand on top of the first one.
- Using a quick, firm, smooth motion, compress the chest three to four inches (less for dogs under 20 pounds), then release.
- Repeat the compressions at a rate of one per second. After every 10 compressions, perform an artificial respiration. Continue this process until veterinary assistance is obtained.

Bleeding

If your pet is bleeding profusely, immediately apply direct pressure to the source of the hemorrhage. Any readily available absorbent material or object including gauze, towels, or shirts, can be used as a compress. Pressure should be applied for no less than five minutes. If bleeding still persists, secure the compress with gauze, a belt, pantyhose, or a necktie and seek veterinary help immediately. If an extremity is involved, apply pressure to the inside, upper portion of the affected leg to reduce blood flow to the limb. If needed, a tourniquet—made with a belt, nectie, or pantyhose—may be applied just above the wound. With a pencil, ruler, or wooden spoon, twist and tighten the tourniquet until bleeding has been minimized. To prevent permanent damage to the limb, be sure you are able to pass one finger between the tourniquet and the skin without too much effort. In addition, release tourniquet pressure for 30 seconds every 10 to 15 minutes, applying direct pressure to the wound during these intervals, until veterinary care is obtained.

Poisonings

General symptoms associated with poisoning include vomiting, diarrhea, unconsciousness, seizures, abdominal pain, excessive salivation, panting, and shock. Common sources of poisoning in older dogs are houseplants, rodent poisons, insecticides, chocolate, ethylene glycol (antifreeze), drug overdose, and ingestion of spoiled or denatured food.

The goal of first aid treatment for poisoning is to dilute or neutralize the poison as much as possible prior to veterinary intervention.

If the poison came from a container, read and follow the label directions concerning accidental poisoning. Be sure to take the label and container with you to your veterinarian. If a label is not available, follow these guidelines:

- If your dog has ingested a caustic or petroleum-based substance or if it is severely depressed, experiencing seizures, or unconscious, waste no time in seeking veterinary help. Treatment in these instances should be administered only under a veterinarian's guidance.
- For other ingested poisons, induce vomiting by administering one teaspoon of hydrogen peroxide per 10 pounds of body weight. Alternatively, use 0.5 milliliter of syrup of ipecac per pound. Repeat the dose of hydrogen peroxide in five minutes, if needed.
- Following evacuation of the stomach, administer two cups of water orally, to help dilute any remaining poison.
- If it is available, administer activated charcoal (mix 25 grams of powder in water to form a slurry, then use 1 milliliter per pound of body weight) or whole milk (1 cup) to help deactivate any residual poison.
- If the poison touched the skin, flush the affected areas with copious amounts of water. If the offending substance is oil-based, use water and a mechanics' hand cleaner or dishwashing liquid to give your pet a quick bath that will remove any remaining residue.
- In all instances of poisoning, specific antidotes may be available at your veterinarian's office. As a result, always seek out professional care following initial first aid efforts.

In an emergency you may face dehydration and circulatory shock, in addition to the conditions discussed above. However, since first aid mea-

Table 14:
At-Home Medications That Can Be Used for First Aid Purposes

If possible, always consult your veterinarian before giving anything orally to your older dog, especially if other medications are currently being given.

Administering oral tablets or capsules: Open your dog's mouth by placing one hand over the top of the muzzle, with your thumb and forefingers placed just behind the upper canine teeth. Slowly tilt your pet's head back, pressing inward and upward with your thumb and forefingers as you go. With your other hand placed at the very front of the lower jaw and holding the pill or capsule, separate the jaws and insert the pill as far back on the tongue as possible. Closing the mouth and lowering the head, gently stroke your pet's throat until you feel a swallow or until your dog licks its nose.

Administering oral liquids: Gently grasp the skin of either cheek and "tent" the skin outward, separating the inner portion of the cheek from the gums. Insert the syringe or spoon containing the medication into the pocket that is formed, then tilt your pet's head slightly upward to prevent the medication from escaping. Gently stroke the neck region until you feel a swallow. Note: Avoid placing liquid medications directly on the back of the tongue or throat; to do so could cause choking.

Medication	Indication	Dosage
3 percent hydrogen peroxide	To induce vomiting General wound cleanser	1 teaspoon per 10 lbs
Bismuth subsalicylate mixtures	Vomiting Diarrhea	1 teaspoon per 20 lbs or 1 tablet per 40 lbs
Buffered aspirin	Fever and inflammation Mild to moderate pain Arthritis	5 to 10 mg per pound every 8 hours (use only on approval by your veterinarian)
Acetaminophen	Same as aspirin	5 mg per pound every 12 hours (use only on approval by your veterinarian)

Table 14 Continued

Medication	Indication	Dosage
Diphenhydramine	Mild cough Allergic reactions	0.5 to 1 mg per pound (use only on approval by your veterinarian)
Kaolin and pectin	Mild diarrhea	Use only under the direction of a veterinarian
Syrup of ipecac	To induce vomiting	1/2 ml per lb
Epsom salts	Constipation; as a soak to reduce swelling and inflammation	For constipation, 1 teaspoon per 10 lbs, dissolved in water and given orally; same dilution for soaks
Milk of magnesia	Vomiting Constipation Deactivate poisons	1 to 2 teaspoons mixed with water
Activated charcoal	Poison deactivation	25 to 50 grams of powder mixed with water; give 1 ml per pound orally
Petroleum jelly	Constipation	1/2 teaspoon per 10 lbs

sures for those two states are limited in scope, only prompt veterinary intervention can save your pet.

Circulatory shock is a life-threatening condition that can result from severe trauma, pain, dehydration, organ malfunction, and the like. With shock, specific physiological reactions impair blood circulation throughout the body and deprive organs and tissues of much-needed oxygen and nutrients. Signs of shock include recumbency; a rapid heart rate; weak pulse; cold, pale mucous membranes; a dry, shrivelled tongue; weakness; panting; subnormal body temperature; and unconsciousness.

Before administering any over-the-counter medications to your dog, consult your veterinarian.

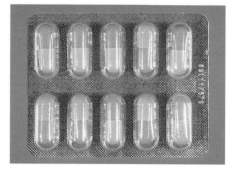

To reverse circulatory shock and preserve life, intravenous fluid and shock medication need to be administered as quickly as possible by a trained veterinarian. At-home first aid should include controlling any predisposing hemorrhage, conserving body temperature by wrapping your pet in a warm towel or blanket, reducing environmental stress, and transporting your dog to the veterinarian as quickly as possible.

Dehydration in dogs is characterized by weight loss, dry gums and mucous membranes, sunken eyeballs, and lethargy. The skin of affected dogs loses its elasticity, as you can tell by gently lifting the skin along the back, then releasing it. If the skin fails to return to its normal position within one second, a state of dehydration exists. As the blood thickens and the organs dehydrate through loss of fluids and electrolytes, circulatory shock and organ failure can ensue.

Some of the instigators of dehydration in older pets are food and water deprivation, burns, bleeding, vomiting, diarrhea, excessive panting, prolonged fever, kidney disease, endocrine disturbances, and certain types of drug therapy.

If you suspect that your pet is dehydrated, seek veterinary care at once. Do not try to treat this condition at home. Only intravenous fluid replacement will effectively reverse the dehydration in a timely manner and lessen or prevent its deleterious effects upon internal organs.

Chapter Seven
Euthanasia and Your Older Dog

With pets living longer than ever before, pet owners need to confront the issue of euthanasia (what it is, how it is performed, and when it is necessary) before it suddenly and unexpectedly confronts them. Although it is an uncomfortable subject, preparing for its possibility will lessen the stress and the guilt you may experience if ever faced with such a decision concerning your devoted companion.

The term euthanasia refers to the purposeful and humane induction of unconsciousness and subsequent death. In veterinary medicine, that is usually accomplished through the use of special injectable formulations of anesthetic agents, such as sodium pentobarbital. Swift and painless, these agents induce death in a matter of seconds.

When does euthanasia become an option? Often, veterinarians are asked to euthanize dogs that are perfectly healthy but possess personality flaws (other than aggressiveness) or physical defects that make them "inconvenient" to their owners. Other dogs are brought in by relatives of a deceased person or of someone who has moved away. They claim that the pet will not be happy with anyone else and that it therefore should be put to sleep. These pets are not candidates for euthanasia, and veterinarians should not be expected to honor such requests. Alternatives do exist, assuming an owner is willing to follow through on the commitment inherent in the initial decision to acquire a pet. It may cost money and time, but that is part of the responsibility.

When legitimate health reasons prompt a responsible pet owner to consider euthanasia, the dog's prognosis and quality of life are factors that enter into the situation. The term prognosis refers to the likelihood of a pet's recovering from an injury, illness, or condition or of its effectively responding to treatment efforts. Pets given a fair to excellent prognosis by a licensed veterinarian are certainly not candidates for euthanasia; they are candidates for treatment. If, on the other hand, the prognosis is poor to grave, then the second factor—quality of life—has to be taken into consideration. Pets that are suffering from a terminal condition yet still have the ability and desire to interact socially with their owners and to eat and drink on their own can be assumed to have an acceptable quality of life. They are not candidates for euthanasia. However, for dogs that do not meet those criteria and for dogs that are experiencing moderate to severe pain on a continual basis—pain that can be effectively relieved only by extra-strength pain relievers—euthanasia should be strongly considered. Please realize that if you are ever faced with such a decision, you will not be alone. Your veterinarian is trained in the euthanasia process and can be trusted to provide you with an accurate prognosis and quality-of-life assessment. That will lead you to a correct decision.

One decision that should be made prior to euthanasia concerns the disposition of the remains. Communal burial sites designated by your city or municipality, private burial sites, including pet memorial parks, and cremation are the three options afforded you. Your veterinarian is knowledgeable about those options and can assist you in making a decision. If you choose a mode of private burial, realize that most cities have laws restricting the burial of animals within city limits. Be sure to check your city code.

Staying with your pet at the time of euthanasia is strictly a matter of preference. If you decide not to be present, rest assured that your pet will experience the comfort and reassurance of gentle, caring hands during these final moments of its life. If you elect to stay by your dog's side during the process, remain as calm as possible so as to avoid upsetting your pet. Gently stroke your dog's head to give it comfort and the reassurance that the suffering will soon be over. Remember, that it is a very stressful and emotional time for your veterinarian as well. Veterinarians went to school to learn how to preserve life, not take it. Few veterinarians can perform this task without sorrow.

The only discomfort a pet may feel during the euthanasia process is caused by the initial insertion of the needle or catheter into the skin and vein. The administration and action of the euthanasia solution itself are painless. Depending upon the mental state and behavior of the pet or upon the degree of its pain from injury or illness, some veterinarians may administer a sedative to calm and relax the patient before it receives the euthanasia solution. Once the euthanasia agent is injected, death takes only seconds. In rare instances, a vocalization or a heavy gasp may be heard as the agent is administered. In addition, evacuation of the bowels and urinary bladder can occur. Pet owners who insist on being present during the euthanasia procedure must realize that these occurrences are not associated with pain or discomfort in any way. These portions of the brain responsible for conscious perception and pain are shut down long before the areas of the brain governing those responses are stimulated by the euthanasia solution. The pet experiences a peaceful, painless, dignified death.

Once the euthanasia procedure is complete, don't hesitate to ask questions and to solicit input from your veterinarian if you are so inclined. Science and research have demonstrated that a strong bond forms between people and their pets. In fact, courses on this human-companion animal bond, the strength of which depends upon numerous relationship factors, are taught in veterinary colleges across the country. It is no wonder that such bonding occurs. The unconditional friendship canine companions provide is difficult to duplicate. They are always there to lend an ear when we need someone to talk to, and regardless of what you may tell them, they still maintain a positive, supporting attitude. Losing such a friend can be quite traumatic, and it is important for us to realize that grieving is a perfectly natural and expected response to the loss of a pet. In our society there is a stigma on grieving openly for a pet that has died or has been put to sleep. However, failure to grieve only causes a buildup of strong emotion and confusion. That is not only psychologically unhealthy, but, as most doctors will point out, physically unhealthy as well. The more you understand about the grieving process and its four stages (denial, anger, depression, acceptance), the quicker the burden of your loss will be lifted. Many excellent books have been written on this subject, and they are readily available at your favorite bookstore or local library.

Pet loss support groups, which exist across the country, can help pet owners endure the loss of a beloved pet. Those groups recognize the strength of the human-companion animal bond and understand its effects during such a difficult time, and that can be quite comforting to a grieving pet owner. To locate support groups near you, contact your veterinarian, the local or state veterinary medical association, the American Veterinary Medical Association, or a local veterinary college. Some veterinary schools have pet-loss counselors on staff ready to assist you in your time of need.

In addition to support groups, many psychologists and psychiatrists in private practice are well trained in pet-loss grieving and support, and they can be called upon to provide one-on-one counseling in such matters. You can usually obtain a list of such specialists from the local or state associations affiliated with those professions.

Donations made in memory of your pet are an excellent means by which you can preserve the precious memory of your faithful companion and at the same time help

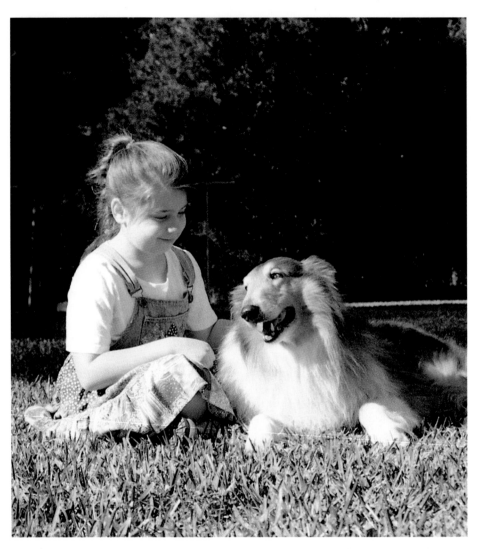

other pets facing the trials of this life. If you would like to establish a memorial fund, contact your local humane society, the local or state veterinary medical association, or the nearest veterinary college. They will be able to assist you in making the proper arrangements.

Glossary

Aberration: Alteration; abnormality.

Abscess: Defined pocket of pus on or within an organ or tissue.

Acariasis: Infestation with mites.

ACTH: Hormone produced by the pituitary gland that regulates steroid production by the adrenal glands.

Acute: (Of clinical disease) brief and severe.

Addison's disease: Disease characterized by insufficient production of steroid hormones by the adrenal glands.

Adenocarcinoma: Malignant tumor involving glandular structures.

Adenoma: Benign tumor involving glandular structures.

ADH: Antidiuretic hormone.

Adrenal glands: Endocrine glands located next to the kidneys that produce, among other things, steroid hormones.

Allergen: Substance capable of producing an allergic response.

Allergy: Exaggerated immune response to some foreign substance.

Alopecia: Hair loss.

ALT (alanine aminotransferase): Liver enzyme.

Anaphylactic reaction: A dramatic fall in blood pressure caused by a massive release of histamine and other chemical within the body.

Anemia: Reduction in the number of red blood cells found within the body.

Anesthesia: Purposeful induction of unconsciousness.

Anorexia: Loss of Appetite.

Antibiotic: Chemical substance capable of killing bacteria or preventing their replication.

Antibodies: Protein structures produced by cells of the immune system that assist in the destruction of foreign organisms and substances.

Antigen: Substance capable of eliciting an immune response.

Antimicrobial: Chemical or substance designed to kill or prevent replication of infectious organisms.

Arrhythmias: Abnormal heartbeats.

Arteries: Vessels that carry blood away from the heart.

Arthritis: Inflammation involving a joint.

Ascarids: Roundworms.

Ascites: Fluid accumulation within the abdominal cavity.

Astringent: Substance that has drying capabilities when applied to a surface.

Atrophy: Shrinking; wasting.

Autoimmune hemolytic anemia: Autoimmune disease characterized by the destruction of red blood cells within the body by the body's own immune system.

Beneficial nematodes: Organisms that, when applied to a yard, will help rid it of flea larvae.

Biopsy: The act of taking an actual tissue sample from an organ or mass and, after proper preparation, examining the tissue microscopically for identification or for the presence of disease.

Bowels: Small and large intestines.

Bromelain: Enzyme supplement used to combat inflammation.

Cachexia: Weight loss, with an overall wasting appearance.

Callus: Region of thickened skin devoid of hair.

Cancer: Malignant neoplasia that spreads into surrounding tissue.

Canine cough complex: Respiratory disease in dogs caused by a group of viral and bacterial organisms that attack the trachea and bronchi and produce inflammation.

Carcinogen: Substance or agent capable of producing neoplastic changes in cells.

Carcinoma: Cancer involving epithelial cells.

Cardiac output: A measure of the heart's ability to pump and circulate blood.

Cardiovascular: Pertaining to the heart and blood vessels.

Cartilage: Sturdy, flexible type of tissue that forms various structures within the body and covers joint surfaces.

Castration: Removal of the testicles.

Cataract: Disease or genetically induced opacity of the lens of the eye.

CBC: Complete blood count.

CCDS: Canine cognitive dysfunction syndrome; senility.

CEHC: Cystic endometrial hyperplasia complex.

Central nervous system: The brain and spinal cord.

Chemotherapy: Treatment of neoplasia by means of chemicals or drugs.

Chronic: (Of clinical disease) having long duration.

Chronic interstitial nephritis: Inflammation of tissue within the kidney.

Chylothorax: Presence of lymph within the chest cavity.

Cirrhosis: Disease characterized by the replacement of healthy tissue with scar tissue.

Coalesce: Combine; consolidate.

Colitis: Inflammation of the colon.

Commercially available: Available over the counter at pet stores, pet supply stores, or veterinary offices.

Congenital disease: Disease condition present, whether noticeable or not, at birth.

COPD: Chronic obstructive pulmonary disease.

Corticosteroids: Chemical compounds produced by the adrenal glands that perform a wide variety of functions within the body; see Glucocorticosteroids.

Cryotherapy: Treatment of neoplasia by means of applications of extreme cold to freeze tumor cells.

Cushing's disease: Disease characterized by overproduction of steroid hormones by the adrenal glands.

Cytology: Diagnostic tool characterized by the microscopic examination and identification of cells taken from fluids, discharges, masses, and tumors.

Definitive diagnosis: A diagnosis that has been confirmed by physical examination or by specific diagnostic tests and procedures.

Dehydration: Condition in which the water level within the body is below that required for normal body functions.

Demarcate: Differentiate; discriminate.

Dermatitis: Inflammation of the skin.

Diagnosis: Identification of the underlying cause of a particular behavior or disease symptom.

DIC: Disseminated intravascular coagulation; formation of small blood clots throughout the body in response to shock or some disease condition.

Dietary indiscretion: The consumption of foodstuffs or substances that are not normal components of a pet's diet.

Diethylcarbamazine: The medication originally used to prevent canine heartworm disease.

Dip: Highly concentrated form of insecticide.

Distemper: Multisystemic disease in dogs caused by a virus.

Diuretic: Drug that moves fluid out of the body by promoting urination.

Dysfunction: Abnormality in function.

ECG: Electrocardiogram; also EKG.

Edema: Fluid retention within the tissues.

Efficacy: Competence; efficiency.

Effusion: Escape of fluid into an open space or cavity.

Electrolyte: Molecule found within the body that is able to conduct electrical current.

Electromyogram: Test used to assess electrical activity within muscle tissue.

Endocrine: Pertaining to glands and hormones within the body.

Endoscope: Instrument used to examine the interior of hollow organs and body cavities.

Enzyme: Chemical substance that enhances and increases the speed of metabolic reactions within the body.

Etiology: Cause of a disease.

Exacerbate: Aggravate; intensify.

Exercise intolerance: Inability to engage in physical exertion without becoming weak or lethargic.

Exorbitant: Excessive; outrageous.

Gastrointestinal: Pertaining to the stomach and intestines.

GDV: Gastric dilatation/volvulus; bloat.

Giardiasis: Intestinal disease caused by a specific protozoal organism.

Gingivitis: Inflammation of the gums.

Glaucoma: Increase in fluid pressure within the eye.

Glucocorticosteroids (Glucocorticoids): One particular class of corticosteroids that is useful in veterinary medicine for the alleviation of inflammation and itching in dogs, as well as the prevention or counteraction of circulatory shock.

Granuloma: Firm mass created by inflammatory cells surrounding a foreign agent or substance.

Halitosis: Bad breath.

Hemoglobin: The molecule found within red blood cells that carries oxygen molecules.

Hemorrhage: Bleeding.

Hemostasis: The ability of the body to control internal or external bleeding.

Hemostatic pathway: Sequence of events that occurs within the body whenever it is called upon to control hemorrhage.

Hepatic: Pertaining to or acting on the liver.

Hernia: Protrusion of an organ or tissue through an unnatural opening.

Hormone: Protein or steroid compound that regulates specific physical and chemical reactions within the body.

Husbandry: Caring for a pet, including feeding, housing, grooming, and preventive health care.

Hybrid vigor: Genetic vitality and strength in offspring resulting from the mating of two purebred dogs of differing breeds.

Hydrophobia: Fear of water.

Hypertrophy: Abnormal enlargement; excessive growth.

Hypoallergenic: Producing very little allergic response.

ICH (infectious canine hepatitis): Viral disease of dogs that adversely affects the liver, kidneys, and other internal organs.

Icterus: Jaundice.

Ictus: True seizure activity.

Idiopathic: Term used to describe any condition for which the cause is unknown.

Immunize: To stimulate an immune response.

Immunotherapy: Treatment of neoplasia by means of immune system components.

Implement: to put into effect; to carry out.

Inappetence: Loss of appetite.

Incapacitate: To disable; to render useless.

Incontinence: The inability to control bodily eliminations.

Inflammation: Bodily response to disease characterized by heat, redness, swelling, and pain.

Innocuous: Harmless; inoffensive.

Insect growth regulator: Chemical substance designed to prevent the development of immature forms of insects into adults.

Insulin: Hormone that regulates the uptake and utilization of glucose within the body.

Integumentary: Pertaining to the skin and associated structures.

Intravenous fluids: Special solutions similar to fluids normally found within the body; used in treatment to correct dehydration and maintain normal water balance within the body and to stimulate cardiac function and blood circulation.

Isoflurane: Type of gas anesthesia commonly selected for use in older pets because of its favorable safety margin.

Ivermectin: Antiparasitic drug that is useful in preventing canine heartworm disease.

KCS: Keratoconjunctivitis sicca.

Keratitis: Inflammation of the cornea.

Ketones: By-products of fat metabolism within the body.

Larva: An immature form of an insect.

Lenticular sclerosis: Cloudiness of the eye lenses occurring as a normal aging change in older dogs.

Leptospirosis: Bacterial disease affecting primarily the kidneys and liver in dogs.

Lethargy: Apathy; listlessness.

Lufenuron: Insect development inhibitor; one of the latest weapons in flea control.

Lumen: The interior of a hollow organ or structure.

Lupus: An autoimmune disease affecting the skin, mucous membranes, and various organs of the body.

Lyme disease: Tick-borne disease causing arthritis and other symptoms in affected hosts.

Lymph: Liquid substance within the body that contains immune cells, proteins, and fat molecules.

Lymphocyte: A type of white blood cell, in some cases capable of producing antibodies.

Malaise: Despondency; weakness.

Malignant: (Of tumor) disposed to grow or spread in frenzied, uncontrolled manner; deadly.

Mange: Infestation with mites.

Metabolism: The sum of all chemical reactions occurring within the body.

Metastasis: The spread of tumor cells from their site of origin to other parts of the body.

Metritis: Inflammation of the uterus.

Microencapsulation: Process by which chemicals, particularly insecticides, are treated to ensure slow, timely, and consistent release of the chemical when applied to the pet or environment.

Microfilariae: Heartworm larvae.

Milbemycin: Drug that is useful in preventing canine heartworm disease.

Musculoskeletal: Pertaining to muscles, bones and joints within the body.

Myelopathy: Degenerative disease of nerve fibers.

Myoglobin: The molecule found within muscle cells that binds oxygen.

Myopathy: Degenerative disease of muscle.

Myositis: Inflammation of muscle tissue.

Neoplasia: Abnormal division and growth of cells within the body.

Neutering: Removal of the ovaries and uterus in the female dog (ovariohysterectomy; spaying) or testicles in the male (castration).

Nidus: Localized area of involvement; source.

Nodular: Round; protruding.

Noxious: Unpleasant; adverse.

Obesity: Disease condition in which excessive amounts of fat exist within the body.

Occult heartworm infection: Heartworm infestation characterized by the presence of adult worms but no circulating larvae.

Omega-3 fatty acids: Fatty acids derived from cold-water fish oil that are used to treat allergies and inflammation in dogs.

Ophthalmic: Pertaining to the eyes.

Organophosphate: Extremely potent (and potentially toxic) class of chemical used in many insecticide products designed for flea and tick control in dogs.

Otitis: Inflammation involving the ear.

Palatability: Taste and flavor appeal of a food.

Palliative: Serving to alleviate without curing.

Palpation: Diagnostic technique used by veterinarians that involves probing and touching of a particular region of the body with the hands and fingers.

Pancreatitis: Inflammation of the pancreas.

Parainfluenza: See Canine cough complex.

Parathyroid glands: Glands closely associated with the thyroid gland in dogs and responsible for regulating levels of calcium within the body.

Parvovirus: Infectious organism that can strike the gastrointestinal system of dogs and cause serious disease.

Pemphigus: Autoimmune skin disease of dogs.

Perineum: The region of the body located between the sexual organs and the anus.

Periodontal disease: Tooth and gum disease.

pH: A measurement used to express the acidity or alkalinity of a solution.

Physiologic: Pertaining to the body, its components, and their functioning.

Pituitary gland: Gland at the base of the brain that produces and stores hormones, most of which control the release of other hormones throughout the body.

Platelet: Blood component that assists in the formation of blood clots.

Pneumothorax: Presence of air within the chest cavity (outside the lungs).

Polydipsia: Increased water consumption.

Polyphagia: Increased appetite.

Polyuria: Increased production and excretion of urine.

Progesterone: Sex hormone responsible for maintaining pregnancy in the female.

Proliferation: Growth; enlargement; production of cells by multiplication of parts.

Prostate gland: Organ at the base of the bladder that surrounds the urethra of males; it produces secretions for semen.

Puberty: Age of sexual maturity.

Pyometra: Condition characterized by pus-filled or fluid-filled uterus.

Pyothorax: Presence of pus within the chest cavity.

Pyrethrin: Relatively safe chemical used in many flea and tick control products.

Rabies: Uniformly fatal viral disease transmitted primarily by the saliva of infected animals.

Radiograph: Pictorial representation of a structure or region of the body created by placing that structure or region over special photographic film and then passing X rays through it.

Regenerative anemia: Anemic condition in which the body is actively replacing the red blood cells that are lost.

Residual: Long-acting; prolonged in effect; remaining.

Retinoids: Vitamin A derivatives used to treat seborrhea in dogs.

Rhinitis: Inflammation of the nasal passages.

Sanguineous: Blood-tinged.

Sarcoma: Malignant neoplasia originating in connective tissue within the body.

Sebaceous gland: Gland attached to a hair follicle that secretes sebum.

Seborrhea: Condition characterized by an abnormal production of skin keratin which causes the skin to crust and scale.

Sebum: Oily secretion of specialized skin glands.

Sedative: Chemical agent that, when administered to a pet, exerts a calming and relaxing effect useful for restraint and minor diagnostic and treatment procedures.

Sensory: Pertaining to vision, hearing, touch, taste, and smell.

Shock (circulatory shock): Life-threatening condition characterized by a gradual shutdown of vital body processes, including blood circulation.

Spay: To remove the ovaries and uterus of a female dog.

Sphincter: Muscular band of tissue that regulates entrance into or exit from an organ.

Stomatitis: Inflammation and infection involving the mouth.

Subcutaneous: Beneath the skin.

Supplement: To add to; enhance.

Symmetry: Balance; congruity.

Syncope: Loss of consciousness caused by oxygen deprivation to the brain.

Tenesmus: Straining to defecate.

Tentative diagnosis: An unconfirmed diagnosis that is usually based upon history, clinical signs, physical examination, and preliminary laboratory findings.

Thoracic: Pertaining to the chest cavity (thorax).

Thorax: The chest cavity.

Thrombocytopenia: Presence of an abnormally low number of platelets within the blood.

Tracheobronchitis: Inflammation of the trachea and bronchi.

Ulcer: An erosion in the lining or surface of an organ.

Ultrasound: The passing of sound waves through the body to create a picture of internal organs and structures on a special screen.

Urethra: Tube-like organ that carries urine from the bladder to the exterior of the body.

Urolith: Mineralized stone within the urinary tract.

Vaccine: A man-made preparation of antigenic substances designed to elicit an immune response when introduced into the body.

Veins: Vessels that carry blood back to the heart.

Vertebrae: Bones composing the spinal column, through which the spinal cord passes.

Vitamin: Organic substance needed for many physiologic processes within the body.

Vitamin K: Vitamin that plays an important role in hemostasis.

X ray: Type of radiation used to obtain a radiograph.

Index

Pancreatic disease, 45
Pancreatitis, 11, 91–92
Parainfluenza, 20
Paralysis, 146–147
Parasites, 8
    external, control of, 23–28
    internal, control of, 21–22
    intestinal, 94–97
Parvovirus, 19
Pemphigus complex, 105
Perianal gland adenomas,
    125–126
Perineal hernia, 75
Periodontal disease, 88–89
Phosphorus, 43
Platelet count, 41
Pleural effusions, 60–61
Pneumonia, 61–62
Pneumothorax, 60–61
Poisonings, 159
Polyphagia, 132
Potassium, 42
Preventive health care, 9–35
Progressive retinal
    atrophy, 110
Prostate disorders, 70
    enlargement, 6
Protein, urine, 47
Pulmonary edema, 60–61
Pyometra, 68–70

Rabies, 20–21
Radiographs, 37–38
Red blood cell count (RBC), 40
Regurgitation, 11; see also
    Vomiting
Reproductive system:
    diagnostic tests, 48
    discharges, 138–140
    diseases of, 68–70
    performance, 6
Respiration, artificial, 157–158
Respiratory system, diseases of,
    58–63
Reticulocyte count, 40
Retinal degeneration, 110–111

Rhinitis, 111–112
Rocky Mountain spotted
    fever, 27
Roundworms, 94

Salivation, excessive, 147
Sebaceous cysts, 8
Seborrhea, 102
Sedation, 34–35
Seizures, 147–149
Selenium, 12–13
Senility, 6, 79–81
"Senior" diets, 10, 14
Sensory functions, aging of,
    107–114
Sertoli cell tumors, 126
Serum creatinine, 42, 64
Shampooing, 26
Shock, 161–162
Skin:
    aging, 7–8
    calluses, 102–103
    diagnostic tests, 49
    diseases of, 98–104
    hair loss, 149–150
    itching, 149–150
    lumps, 150–151
Smell, sense of, 111–112
    loss of, 112
Sneezing, 151
Sodium, 10, 42
Spinal column, 6–7
    disk disease, 76–78
Spondylosis deformans, 72
Squamous cell carcinomas, 126
Stranguria, 153
Sudden acquired retinal
    degeneration (SARD), 110
Swelling, facial, 141
Swimming, 15–16
Symptoms, 130–156

Table scraps, feeding, 11–12
Tapeworms, 23, 95–96
Temperature, 17
Tenesmus, 134–135

Thirst, excessive, 151–152
Ticks, 8, 24, 27–28
Tobacco smoke, 4, 17
Toenails, 7
Total serum protein, 43
Trachea, collapsed, 59–60
Tracheobronchitis, 59
Travel, 16–17
Tumors, see Cancer

Ulcers, 89–90
Ultrasonography, 38
Urinalysis, 46–47
Urinary system:
    diagnostic tests, 48
    diseases of, 63–68
    incontinence, 5–6
    infections, 65–67
    infections, 65–67
    stones, 67–68, 153
Urination:
    excessive, 152
    incontinence, 152–153
    straining, 153
Urine:
    sediment, 47
    tests, 37
Urolithiasis, 11, 67–68

Vaccinations, 18–21
Vestibular disease, 78–79
Vision, see Eyes
Vitamin K, 57–58
Vitamin supplements, 12
Vomiting, 11, 154–155

Water, 12
Weakness, 155
Weight loss, 155–156
White blood cell:
    serum, 41
    differentiation and
        percentages, 41
    urine, 47

Zinc, 12

"A solid bet for first-time pet owners"
—*Booklist*

We've taken all the best features of our popular Pet Owner's Manuals and added *more* expert advice, *more* sparkling color photographs, *more* fascinating behavioral insights, and fact-filled profiles on the leading breeds. Indispensable references for pet owners, ideal for people who want to compare breeds before choosing a pet. Over 120 illustrations per book – 55 to 60 in full color!

"Stunning"
– Roger Caras
Pets & Wildlife

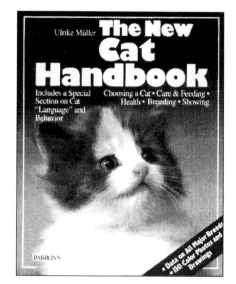

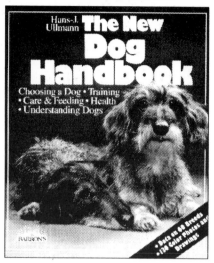

THE NEW AQUARIUM HANDBOOK, Scheurmann (3682-4)
THE NEW AUSTRALIAN PARAKEET HANDBOOK, Vriends (4739-7)
THE NEW BIRD HANDBOOK, Vriends (4157-7)
THE NEW CANARY HANDBOOK, Vriends (4879-2)
THE NEW CAT HANDBOOK, Müller (2922-4)
THE NEW CHAMELEONS HANDBOOK, Le Berre (1805-2)
THE NEW COCKATIEL HANDBOOK, Vriends (4201-8)
THE NEW DOG HANDBOOK, H.J. Ullmann (2857-0)
THE NEW DUCK HANDBOOK, Raethel (4088-0)
THE NEW FINCH HANDBOOK, Koepff (2859-7)
THE NEW GOAT HANDBOOK, Jaudas (4090-2)
THE NEW PARAKEET HANDBOOK, Birmelin / Wolter (2985-2)
THE NEW PARROT HANDBOOK, Lantermann (3729-4)
THE NEW RABBIT HANDBOOK, Vriends-Parent (4202-6)
THE NEW SALTWATER AQUARIUM HANDBOOK, Blasiola (4482-7)
THE NEW SOFTBILL HANDBOOK, W. Steinigeweg (4075-9)
THE NEW TERRIER HANDBOOK, Kern (3951-3)

Barron's Educational Series, Inc.
250 Wireless Blvd., Hauppauge, NY 11788
In Canada: Georgetown Book Warehouse
34 Armstrong Ave., Georgetown, Ont. L7G 4R9
Barron's ISBN prefix: 0-8120   (#63) R3/96
Order from your favorite bookstore or pet shop.

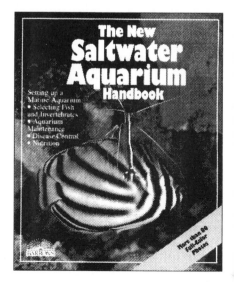